....

BANISH BLOATING

Also by Suzannah Olivier

. . . .

What Should I Feed My Baby?

The Breast Cancer Prevention and Recovery Diet

The Stress Protection Plan

Also in the *You Are What You Eat* series

. . . .

Natural Hormone Balance

Maximising Energy

Suzannah Olivier

BANISH

BLOATING

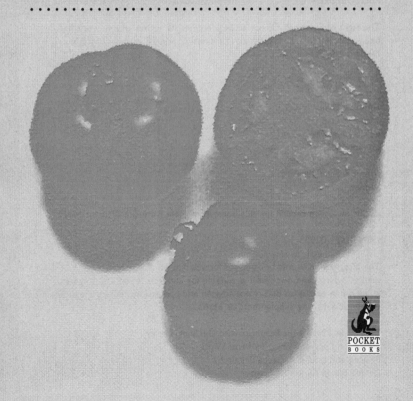

POCKET
BOOKS

First published in Great Britain by Pocket Books, 2000
An imprint of Simon & Schuster UK Ltd
A Viacom Company

10 9 8 7 6 5 4 3 2 1

Simon & Schuster UK Ltd
Africa House
64-78 Kingsway
London WC2B 6AH

Simon & Schuster Australia
Sydney

A CIP catalogue record for this book is available from the British Library

ISBN 0-671-02953-3

The information in this book is not intended as an alternative to
medical advice, and none of it is suitable for children. If you are pregnant,
going on an exclusion diet is not advised and professional advice must be
sought about using supplements or herbs.

Typeset in 12 on 14pt Perpetua with Gill Sans display
Design and page make-up by Peter Ward
Printed and bound in Great Britain by
Omnia Books Limited, Glasgow

This book is dedicated to G.E.E.

Contents

PART SIX

HEALING WITH E.A.S.E

PART SEVEN

APPENDICES

Part One

THE BLOATING

BLUES

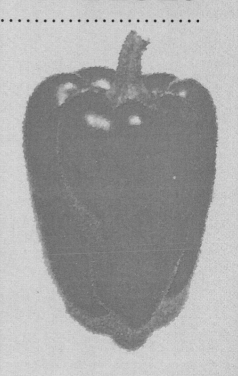

CHAPTER ONE

Introduction

Look up bloating in most medical textbooks and you will find it doesn't exist. Various related conditions might satisfy your search for information – oedema, flatulence, colic – but not bloating. And yet 70 per cent of women who seek help from nutritionists, and 40 per cent of men, note that bloating is a feature, or the core, of their health problems.

When bloating is acknowledged as a problem by the medical profession it is usually viewed as 'idiopathic' – caused by unknown factors – and nothing in the doctor's little black bag can help long term. Diuretics or indigestion remedies may be prescribed for a while, but these will only deal with the symptoms, and not address the underlying causes. In the meantime a fortune is spent on these medications, both prescribed and over-the-counter.

Very few people like to bother their doctors with this problem in the first place – even though there now appears to be an epidemic of bloating. This non-specific term can be, and has been, applied to a variety of symptoms, many of which, for some reason, also begin with the letter B – burping, belching, blimping, bubbling, ballooning, billowing, bursting, bulging. From 'football tummy' to 'banana fingers', bloating causes much daily misery. It is not unusual for people to have morning clothes and afternoon clothes, which allow for an extra few centimetres of girth. Shoes may be bought in two sizes for good days and bad days. Whole suitcases are carried under eyes. Breasts may take on a life of their own for two, or more, weeks out of a four-week cycle. Wedding rings are discarded, not due to divorce, but to swollen fingers. Bloating can involve an uncomfortable, distended feeling that does not seem to be related to any particular cause, and also trapped wind which seems to have no pattern. Slim people can have the most extraordinarily swollen tummies, which go up and down with the hours of the day.

Bloating may be involved in gaining excess weight – though it has got nothing to do with gaining excess fat. It can, however, have a lot to do with water retention. It is easy to mistake water retention for gaining fat weight, but the way to tell if it is water retention is quite easy. If when you go on a weight-reduction diet, or follow a 'detox' plan, you lose several kilograms within a week or two then this is water retention – we can only realistically lose a maximum of a kilogram of fat-weight in any given week. If you press your finger into an area of the body which feels swollen, for instance hands or feet, and find that an indentation remains after taking your finger away, then this is water retention. If the weight gained fluctuates depending on the time of the day, the time of the month or even the time of the year, it is water retention.

SYSTEM OVERLOAD

We overload ourselves daily in our high-tech, fast-paced world, and bloating is a major symptom of overload on our health. Because it is not life threatening it is easy to just accept bloating as one of life's trials, or even to ignore it. For many people bloating is a symptom which is sufficiently irritating to want to do something about it, if only they knew what, while for others it is more debilitating and interferes with their enjoyment of daily life. It can lead to cutting back on social activities and sports, as well as days off work.

No symptom, even if it seems minor, should be ignored if it persists. Bloating on a regular basis can be indicative of underlying health issues and imbalances which, if left unchecked and untreated, can lead to more serious health problems in later years. The good news is that, because we are a complex web of interactions, it is impossible to positively affect one aspect of health without influencing other aspects. This is why someone who deals with their bloating and digestive problems, even minor ones, may find that other health issues, such as migraines, asthma, eczema and arthritis, resolve themselves. If you experience bloating, you are probably receiving an early warning signal that all is not well and something needs to be addressed to ensure long-term health. Quite a thought! You imagined you were just working out why your trousers no longer fastened, but you may actually be keeping diseases at bay. Hippocrates knew that digestive health was important when he wrote in around 400 BC, 'Death sits in the bowels, and bad digestion is the root of all evil'.

CHAPTER TWO

Earth, Fire, Wind and Water

If you are lucky, the bloating you are experiencing may be quite a simple issue which can be resolved by addressing one or two dietary factors. If the situation is more complex, perseverance may be needed to uncover the underlying cause.

The factors which contribute to bloating can be varied. One way of remembering the likely causes of bloating is to link them to the four elements: Earth, Fire, Wind and Water.

EARTH

One hundred trillion bacteria reside in our digestive tracts and we have ten times more bacteria in, and on, our bodies than we have cells. About 400–500 of these bacteria species live in our bowels and they are major players in the bloating story (see Wind below). In a garden the bacterial balance of the earth is known to be vital to the health of the plants growing in that soil. The minute that you start spraying chemicals, using artificial fertilisers, or if you grow the same crop in the same patch year-in year-out, you begin to change the bacterial balance of the soil. In much the same way, when we eat certain foods in quantity we change the make-up of the bacteria in our guts. The earth element, or bacterial balance, is one of the most important factors to address when contending with bloating and we will be talking about it in detail.

FIRE

This element is a good analogy for inflammation, which is one of the main factors associated with the problem of bloating, general digestive discomfort and a host of specific digestive problems – gastritis, colitis, diverticulitis. The suffix 'itis' just means inflammation, and you can guarantee that if a condition needs to be called an itis, then it is already quite serious. However, most people carry on with their daily lives, suffering with bloating and other digestive problems unaware that inflammation is a major player in their health. Inflammation is characterised by redness, soreness and inflamed or bloated tissues. The inflamed area is evidence of our immune systems mounting a defence against irritants such as certain foods, toxic by-products of bacteria, or 'foreign bodies' such as viruses and parasites. Tackling the condition early is obviously ideal, and much can be done to reverse the situation and put out the fire in your gut.

WIND

The subject of many jokes, wind causes a lot of discomfort and, for some people, significant embarrassment. It is a major cause of bloating. Burping, flatulence, trapped wind, gurgling sounds, distended tummies – all are signs of wind which is brewing up a storm in one part of our digestive tract or another. Men and women can suffer equally from 'windy' problems. It is normal to 'break wind' at the rate of 100 mph and this is not, with a healthy digestive tract, offensive. Wind, or 'flatus' is comprised of more than 250 different gases, and the study of flatulence is called flatology. It is a serious science: one scientific paper described 'flatoanalysis, airflow studies and flatulograms'.

A certain amount of air can be swallowed and may contribute to the problem, but the main cause is likely to be fermentation. A number of aspects of our diet can predispose us to having a gas factory in our digestive tracts. When anything is fermented, for example beer or wine, gas is produced by the actions of sugar and yeast. In some beers, and in champagne, gas is trapped in the bottle giving a good analogy for what happens in the gut. The degree of gassiness or 'head' that you will find in a beer is dependent upon the type of yeast used, how much sugar it contains and how long it is fermented. If digestion is impaired and starches and sugars are not broken down adequately into simple sugars, gas is the result.

Other aspects of our diet can contribute to this volatile problem being above and beyond what might be considered normal, and manipulation of our diet can significantly ease, or totally eliminate, the problem of excess wind.

WATER

Water retention is another major form of bloating. It is frequently suffered by women, though men are not immune to the problem. Two principal reasons seem to be behind water retention, and they can be loosely categorised as toxic build-up and hormonal imbalances.

Toxic build-up can come from a number of sources – we are exposed to many sources of chemicals in our environment. Those that are found in our food include preservatives, colours, flavour enhancers, pesticides, herbicides and fertilisers. A significant amount of food toxins comes from eating foods to which we are allergic or sensitive. While these foods may not be universally toxic, people can have individual reactions which contribute to their overall toxic load. Many people also tend to drink dehydrating drinks, such as tea, coffee and alcohol, which can contribute to the problem of toxin overload.

Water is the means by which toxic substances can be

diluted to the point where they are unable to do harm. In its wisdom, if the body is overloaded with toxins that it cannot eliminate, it will seek to neutralise them by surrounding them with water molecules. This build-up of surplus water leads to water retention.

A contributing factor to water retention can be hormone imbalances, especially of female hormones. One of the main female hormones, oestrogen, plumps out tissues, which contribute to the female shape. But when too much oestrogen is being produced, the plumping process is increased, and this can lead to water retention, especially in areas such as breasts, and particularly nearer to the 'time of the month'. The key factors that affect bloating of any sort, including hormonal bloating, are diet, digestive health, and food allergies and intolerances. In particular, if there is insufficient fibre in the diet, oestrogens are forced to re-circulate in the body, and make the problem worse.

Part Two

EAT YOUR FOOD

(DON'T LET IT

EAT YOU!)

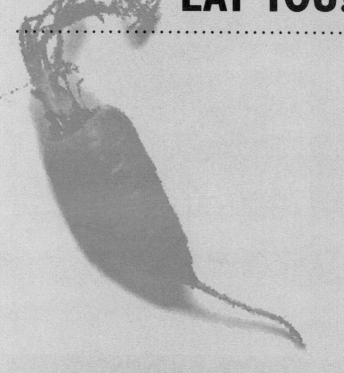

CHAPTER THREE

Introduction

. . . .

In order to understand why we get bloated it is worth going on a trip around your inner tube – your digestive tract – to find out what happens. Before we do go on this tour, it helps to first understand the basics of what different groups of food do to enable us to maintain optimal health, and how they can also be the source of problems. Foods have to be broken down to their smallest components in order to be friend, and not foe. Technically, these molecules remain 'outside' the body until they are absorbed across the gut wall and into the bloodstream, where they are sent on their journey to be used for building and repair jobs as well as for fuel. Food molecules can be immensely disruptive to the workings of the body and may set up allergy reactions if they are not fully digested into a form that is useful. If the food is not broken down properly, and if the digestive tract is weakened and 'leaky', the incompletely digested food molecules can be absorbed.

These days, social gatherings are fraught with dietary minefields. Some people spend much of the time dodging around the many foods to which they have attributed their bloating problems, while desperately trying to not draw attention to themselves. Is their behaviour necessary? Is it based on unfounded phobias? Or on facts?

While many people are certain that the food they are eating is a culprit, they are unable to pinpoint precisely what they need to avoid. This is hardly surprising when there is uncertainty about the components of the foods we buy, and how, where and why we digest food. This chapter, and the next, aims to pour light on these subjects.

Ideally, it is best to approach the question of food in a positive way. Instead of worrying about the foods that you are not 'permitted', I would suggest that you focus on the many foods that you are able to eat. You will find, in the chapter **Healing with E.A.S.E.**, page 97, lists of foods to stock in your cupboards and fridge which you will be able to eat without worry. There are also some suggested eating plans. This chapter also looks at ways to repair your system in order that foods which you may currently need to avoid can be reintroduced at a later stage. By all means find the culprit, if indeed there is one, and understand the importance of good nutrition, but remember: Enjoy your food. Eat for nourishment, energy and pleasure. Food is one of our greatest sensory delights and is vital for positive health.

FOOD FACTS

The main components of our food are proteins, fats and carbohydrates. Along with the vitamins and minerals, some of these are termed 'essential' while the remainder are non-essential. There are around 47 essential nutrients which we can only obtain from our diet because our bodies are unable to manufacture them, and these are amino acids (protein building blocks), certain fatty acids, vitamins and minerals. All of these nutrients are the essential parts of the jigsaw puzzle which allows functions to happen in every cell. If a part of the jigsaw puzzle is missing then the picture cannot be completed.

The most concentrated source of vitamins and minerals in the diet are fruits, vegetables, pulses, nuts, seeds, cereals, moderate amounts of dairy products and moderate amounts of meat and fish, though a well-balanced vegetarian diet is unlikely to be deficient in nutrients for most people. The weakest, or most depleted, source of nutrients are processed foods, sugar, refined grains and alcohol.

But a nutrient-rich diet is not always sufficient if there has been a history of poor diet or if illness has been experienced. Frequently, digestion has been impaired to such an extent that food is not being efficiently broken down to release the nutrients, or the lining of the digestive tract is not adequately absorbing them. This means that digestive health must be restored before a full return to health can be experienced.

CHAPTER FOUR

Building Blocks

. . . .

Before we go on a tour of the digestive tract, we will look briefly at the effects that the various food components have on health and bloating. In the main we use carbohydrates for fuel, while proteins and fats are turned into building materials for the body.

PROTEINS

They are used to build all the solid structures – bones, teeth, hair, nails – as well as the soft tissues – the cells of all the organs, skin and blood. They also make up the internal chemicals and messengers which allow us to function – hormones, enzymes and nerve chemicals.

Proteins in our diet are found in animal products – meat, cheese, milk and eggs – but hardly at all in the fatty animal products such as butter or cream. They are also found in many plant sources such as nuts, seeds, legumes (pulses, beans, peas), grains (cereals, bread, rice), quinoa, and in small amounts in most vegetables and fruits.

Proteins are broken down in our digestive tract into their smallest components, amino acids. These can then be carried across the gut wall and into our blood streams. They are then taken to the liver, where the amino acids are linked together again to make up the structural and chemical proteins of which we are composed.

We need protein. It is the key building block in our body and insufficient amounts can lead to a number of degenerative diseases. However, deficiency is mainly a problem of undeveloped countries where there are variable food supplies, poor nutritional education and, in the worst cases, famine. In the West we have the opposite problem and we tend to get too much protein in our diet.

How proteins affect bloating

Some people find that protein foods are best not eaten with carbohydrate foods and that in so doing they can significantly reduce their bloating problems, see **Stop Foods Fighting**, page 129. Proteins can often interfere with the digestion of carbohydrates, or vice versa. It is also suspected that the protein content of some grains – the gluten components – prevent their proper breakdown in some people, resulting in health problems, including bloating.

An excess of animal protein in particular has been linked to the explosion – forgive the pun – of gas problems which plague some people with bloating. To put it bluntly, if the gas you expel smells unpleasant then the chances are that you are eating too much animal protein or not digesting it properly. The reason for this is that animal proteins contain high levels of smelly sulphur. (Sulphur is also one of the most widely used preservatives and is present in a majority of processed foods. Everything from instant potato, to jam, dried fruit, wine, beer and cider.)

In summary, proteins can cause bloating-related problems when they are not broken down properly – either because the digestive mechanism is not working properly, or because too much protein is being consumed.

FATS

Fats can be divided into two categories: those that are vital for health and those that do not actively support good health, and can even be damaging.

The good guys Structural fats are the most important because without them we would suffer a number of deficiency diseases. They are used both as building blocks for cell membranes in the skin and in the organs, and for building nervous tissue. They are also the basis of hormone production. They are unsaturated fats and are found in vegetables, and in nuts and seeds and their oils (e.g. sunflower, walnut and sesame oils). Another key source of these valuable unsaturated fats is oily fish, such as tuna, sardines, mackerel, salmon, pilchards and anchovies. Some of the fats that make up this group are called essential fats, because they are, literally, essential to our health – we cannot manufacture them and we must obtain them from our diet.

The not-so-good guys The storage fats provide warmth and energy reserves for future needs. They also provide the padding that protects our internal organs and lies on our hips and waists. They are saturated fats and are mainly found in animal products – meat, milk, cheese, cream and eggs. It is not essential to include saturated fats in our diet because we can make this type very easily by converting carbohydrates – so it is not necessary to eat fat to become fat!

The downright awful A class of fats that could also come under the same heading as saturated fats are the hydrogenated, or trans-fats. These are man-made fats found in margarines and in packaged foods such as pies, pasties, biscuits, crisps and chocolates. While these originate from vegetable or seed oils, causing many people to believe them to be healthy, they have been chemically altered to behave like saturated fats. Thus, all that is good about these oils has been destroyed. They also have added health hazards as they are a source of free-radicals, unstable molecules which can damage body tissues. Vegetable oils can also harbour trans-fats if they have been allowed to go rancid, if they have been extracted by chemical means, left open to light and heat, or are used for cooking.

For this reason it is best to buy cold-pressed oils, to keep them in the fridge and use them on salads or as dressings for cooled vegetables. The best fats for cooking, which are not so readily damaged, are olive oil, coconut butter or a little ordinary butter from time to time.

How fats affect bloating

Excess animal fats in the diet encourage inflammation by encouraging an inflammatory substance called PGE2, and if this inflammation happens in the digestive tract, this can contribute to a sensation of bloating. On the other hand, the healthy fats, found in vegetables, nuts, seeds, their oils, and in oily fish, encourage two anti-inflammatory substances called PGE1 and PGE3 and these substances have the power to heal gut tissue. Finally, hydrogenated fats block the effects of the beneficial anti-inflammatory PGE1 and PGE3 and so contribute to bloating.

Another important aspect to consider is that fat in the diet is how we obtain the fat-soluble vitamins A, D, E and K. Of particular interest are vitamins A and E; both are antioxidant vitamins, and vitamin A is essential for tissue repair. Antioxidants help to reduce damage to the digestive tract when there is inflammation and to repair the tissue. Vitamin A deficiency commonly manifests itself as mouth ulcers and poor healing of tissues. This is usually replicated internally – you just can't see it.

CARBOHYDRATES

Carbohydrates provide our main source of energy. Understanding the basic structure of different carbohydrates is helpful in getting to grips with why sugars and carbohydrates can cause so many problems with bloating in sensitive people. If the carbohydrates are not broken down properly into 'single' sugars they can be acted upon by 'unfriendly' bacteria in the intestines and bowels.

The simplest components of carbohydrates are saccharides – which just means sugars. How many saccharides there are, and how they are joined together dictates the type of carbohydrate they make. Their structure also determines how fast these saccharides, or sugars, are delivered into the blood, and therefore how speedily they deliver energy.

Slow-releasing carbohydrates are best for us as they deliver a constant source of fuel which does not stress our systems with peaks and troughs of energy. The slow-releasing carbohydrates are found in starches, or complex carbohydrates. Sources of these include wholemeal bread, whole grain brown rice, potato jackets, brown pasta, sweet potatoes, whole porridge oats and muesli. Most vegetables (other than cooked root vegetables) also provide a slow-releasing source of energy, but they are not concentrated sources of complex carbohydrates as they have a high water and fibre content. The fibre found in slow-releasing carbohydrates is highly beneficial for digestive health and for bringing bloating under control.

Fast-releasing carbohydrates have a more immediate effect on glucose in the blood, which can be stressful for the body to adapt to. Fast-releasing carbohydrates are in the simple sugars found in table sugar, confectionery, biscuits, cakes, crisps, white bread, white rice, many processed breakfast cereals, potatoes without their skins (as in mashed potato or chips), and many cooked root vegetables (e.g. carrots, parsnips, beetroot). Single-sugar carbohydrates are found in fruit, but the fibre content and the form in which these sugars are found (fructose) moderates their impact and makes them a healthy option. Fast-releasing carbohydrates, apart from most fruits, have the effect of feeding bacteria in the bowels, and favouring the proliferation of 'bad' bacteria which contribute significantly to bloating in all its forms – wind, inflammation, water retention and hormonal balance.

Types of sugars and starches

As carbohydrates are one of the main culprits in the bloating story, it is helpful to have a basic understanding of the different types, where they are found, and how they are digested.

1. **Single sugars** Glucose (also called Dextrose), Fructose, Galactose

   Single sugars are called monosaccharides ('mono' meaning one, so one-sugar), and they do not need to be digested for them to be taken across the gut wall into the blood-stream.

   Where to find them
   Glucose – Honey, fruits, some vegetables.
   Fructose – Fruits, honey, some vegetables.
   Galactose – Yoghurt that is home-made and fermented for at least 24 hours.

2. **Double sugars** Lactose, Sucrose, Maltose, Isomaltose

   These sugars are called disaccharides ('di' meaning two, so two-sugars). They need to be split into single sugars by digestive enzymes in the gut in order for them to pass across the gut wall. Each sugar has a specific enzyme that acts upon it. If this particular enzyme is lacking this can contribute significantly to bloating. For example, if someone is deficient in the milk sugar splitting enzyme, lactase, the milk sugar in dairy products, lactose, can cause problems for that person.

Where to find them

Lactose – Milk, milk powder, commercial yoghurt,
home-made yoghurt fermented for less than 24 hours
processed cheeses, cottage cheese, cream cheese, ice
cream, whey; also some drugs and nutritional
supplements (read the labels).

Sucrose – Table sugar (whether white or brown), molasses,
treacle, golden syrup, dark sugars. Sucrose is also added
to many processed foods, such as desserts, ketchup,
canned foods, cereals, etc.

Maltose and Isomaltose – Corn syrup, malted milk, sweets,
products using corn syrup (e.g. banana chips). Most of
the maltose and isomaltose found in the digestive tract is
the result of partially digested starches (polysaccharides),
which are meant to be broken down into simple sugars.
Isomalt is also added as a bulk sweetener to some
commercial foods.

3. **Starches** Amylose, Amylopectin

Also called polysaccharides ('poly' meaning many, so
many-sugars). Most vegetables, especially root vegetables, grains, beans and pulses contain both of these two
starches, in different ratios. The different proportions of
these two types of starch may influence the relative
digestibility of various starch-bearing foods for people
with differing digestive capabilities. If any of the digestive
steps do not take place efficiently, resistant starch
molecules and disaccharides remain in the intestines to
increase bacterial fermentation. It has been estimated
that up to 20 per cent of bread starch, for instance, is not
broken down in some people. Additionally, more
modified starch is creeping into our food packets and

those with a sensitivity need to be wary.

4. **Fibre**

This is the indigestible component of starchy foods. Fibre can be soluble or insoluble and we need both types to maintain the health of the digestive tract. Though fibre is not digested by the human digestive tract, it provides bulk for it to 'work on', regulates the passage of stools and provides a source of energy for 'good' bacteria in the bowels. All plant foods contain fibre in different proportions, however refined foods, such as white bread, white rice, the flesh of cooked potatoes, and packaged convenience foods, such as crisps and biscuits, contain low amounts of fibre. For more information about fibre see Fab Fibre, page 166.

5. **Other sugars**

Sorbitol, Xylitol These are sugars which cannot be digested by the human body and so they are used by food manufacturers in diabetic jams and other foods. Because they are labelled 'sugar-free', many people avoiding sugars will use these products, even if they are not diabetics. Large amounts of these sugars cause gas and bloating, but even small amounts can be a problem for sensitive people. The diarrhoea associated with these sweeteners is referred to as 'Halloween diarrhoea', because a favourite joke is to give sorbitol-based candy to trick-or-treaters.

CHAPTER FIVE

Gluttons for Gluten

The foods that we are most likely to be sensitive to are those to which we are well and truly addicted. And high up the list of those foods are bread, pasta and other wheat-based products. 'I couldn't have a meal without some bread', 'I don't know what to have if I don't have a sandwich for lunch at work', 'I just love pasta and eat it three times a week – it is so easy to cook', these are common sentiments. But wheat-based foods are high in gluten, as are those made with the grains oats, rye and barley.

Gluten is a sticky molecule which traps air in the bread-making process – a very useful characteristic, as it ensures loaves puff up nicely and are springy to the touch. It is this feature that is particularly appealing to bakers. Bread is sold by volume and not by weight, so the more a loaf puffs up, the less the ingredients cost, and the more profitable it becomes. Because of this, many large commercial bakeries have encouraged the development of strains of wheat which provide these qualities more successfully. This means that modern strains have been bred to contain even more gluten, and this seems to be contributing to the increase in gluten intolerance. To add to this problem, wheat is an inexpensive ingredient which, as modified starch, is used to bulk out many convenience foods, meaning that we are exposed to gluten more often that we realise. As a result, it is hard to find commercially produced, processed foods on the supermarket shelves which are wheat free.

COELIAC DISEASE

The orthodox view of gluten allergy is that it is only suffered by those with confirmed coeliac disease, where the gluten is responsible for 'wearing down', or atrophying the villi in the digestive tract. The villi are microscopic finger-like protrusions which line our digestive tracts and increase the area of absorption. They also secrete the digestive enzymes which break down carbohydrates. Because the villi are atrophied, the intestine is unable to perform its job of secreting these enzymes, and it is also unable to satisfactorily absorb the nutrients which have been successfully digested.

GLUTEN GRAIN INTOLERANCE

Coeliac disease is not, however, the whole story, and many people may have a number of the same symptoms without the definitive damage to their villi that is suffered by true coeliacs. In some way the gluten is affecting their digestive tract sufficiently to impair digestion and to cause wide ranging digestive symptoms, including bloating, abdominal cramping, diarrhoea and gas. Other more general symptoms include low energy, sluggish metabolism, allergies, skin problems and headaches, and many people find these can be resolved by addressing gluten grain intolerance.

It seems likely that one of the reasons why gluten grains are a problem for a significant number of people is that the grains trigger an immune reaction which causes no immediate damage to the villi, but which ultimately causes inflammation and leads to increased gut permeability. This can lead to many of the symptoms described. For a full description of increased gut permeability see Help! I've Sprung a Leak, page 61.

Because these people are not 'true' coeliacs this does not mean that their symptoms are to be discounted, as is sometimes suggested. What it probably means is that we do not yet have sensitive enough tests to fully establish what the 'biochemical' reason for their symptoms is. What we can do, however, is to experiment by avoiding gluten grains, and, in a few cases, other carbohydrate sources, to establish if their problems are being caused by these.

TROPICAL SPRUE

A third problem associated with gluten is tropical sprue. This is caused by an infection or toxin which, as the name implies, is more likely to be acquired when a person is exposed to unfamiliar climates and environments. It results in disruption of the villi in such a way that it mimics coeliac disease. Once it has been treated with antibiotics, gluten grains can be reintroduced.

GLUTEN CONTAINING FOODS

Generally speaking, people with coeliac disease will need to avoid gluten grains for their entire lives, while people with gluten-grain intolerance may be able to reintroduce gluten grains after a period of time (usually six to 12 months), though probably in reduced quantities and on a rotation basis. Those with tropical sprue will probably be able to reintroduce gluten containing foods without problems after their antibiotic treatment is completed.

- Grains containing gluten are wheat (which has the highest amount of gluten and is therefore the most troublesome), oats, rye, barley, tricale and spelt.
- Common wheat containing foods include breads, pasta, pastry, breakfast cereals and mueslies, couscous, bulgar, biscuits, cakes, foods in batter or breadcrumbs, semolina.

Gluten-free versions of many of these foods are available at health food shops, and gluten-free baking cookbooks are readily available, see **Resources**, page 198.

● Grains which do not contain gluten are rice, millet, quinoa (not technically a grain, but used like one), corn (though it is the most common cause of grain intolerance in the USA), and buckwheat (which is not the same family as wheat, despite the name).

● Foods which may contain hidden gluten include TVP (textured vegetable protein), barley malt, starch other than cornstarch (i.e. modified starch in an ingredients listing), maltodextrin, ice creams with gluten stabilisers, processed meats (sausages, luncheon meats) and some processed cheeses containing wheat flour or oat gum. If you are highly sensitive to gluten then also check the following for their full ingredients: curry powder, white pepper, dry seasoning mixes, gravy mixes, chutneys and other condiments, ketchup, dips, chewing gum, pie fillings, baked beans, baking powder, salad dressings, sandwich spreads, instant coffee, chocolates, vanilla and flavourings made with alcohol.

CHAPTER SIX

Doubts about Dairy

While we think of dairy products as protein foods, they can cause great problems for people who are sensitive to the milk sugar, or carbohydrate, lactose.

We produce a specific enzyme, lactase, which digests milk sugar. If lactose is not properly digested then, as with any sugar, it can be fermented by the bacteria in the gut and produce uncomfortable bloating. Babies are born with the ability to digest milk, as they are meant to be breastfed, however in a significant number of people the production of lactase tails-off from the age of around two or three. In addition to severe wind and bloating, other signs of lactose intolerance can include constipation, diarrhoea, excess mucus production, ulcerative colitis and IBS (irritable bowel syndrome).

LACTOSE – MILK'S SWEET REVENGE

Lactose intolerance varies in adults of different ethnic backgrounds, and the lactase enzyme is significantly absent in some racial groups. The percentage of people of Jewish, Mediterranean, African, Hispanic, Asian and Native American descent who are lactose intolerant varies between 65–95 per cent, whereas only 10–15 per cent of those of Northern or Middle European descent are lactose intolerant.

Not all dairy products are rich sources of lactose and so some dairy foods are tolerated by lactose-intolerant adults, where others are not. For instance, the processing of milk into cheese will remove most of the milk sugars, leaving behind the protein and fat, and butter is almost 100 per cent fat with little residual lactose. Yoghurt, home-made and fermented for 24 hours, is yet another exception as the bacteria which is used in the manufacturing process largely pre-digests the milk sugars. Skimmed milk will have a higher amount of lactose, compared to full fat milk, and can cause greater problems for sensitive individuals.

High lactose foods – 4+ g per 100 g/ml of product
   cow's milk, skimmed
   cow's milk, semi-skimmed
   cream, single
   fromage frais
   goat's milk
   marscapone
   quark
   sheep's milk
   whey milk
   yoghurt, low-fat and full fat, cow's
   yoghurt, sheep's and goat's

Medium lactose foods – 1–4 g per 100 g/ml of product
   cheese, cottage
   cheese, ricotta
   cow's milk, full fat
   cream, double
   crème fraîche
   yoghurt, Greek, cow's

Low lactose foods – less than 1 g per 100 g/ml of product
   butter
   cheese, hard (Cheddar, Parmesan)
   cheese, soft (Brie)

ghee
lactose-free milk (from which lactose has been removed)

Lactose intolerance can be tested for by rigorously avoiding lactose containing foods for a two-week period to see if any symptoms, such as bloating, excess mucus or diarrhoea, improve. If they worsen again after reintroducing lactose you can assume that this is at least a part of the problem.

MILK PROTEINS

The other constituents of milk which cause problems in sensitive people are milk proteins, and the most troublesome of the proteins is casein. Milk proteins can cause a straightforward allergy reaction or can create a more subtle sensitivity. Either way they can irritate the gut lining, which can exacerbate inflammation, which in turn can increase bloating.

Another recently identified problem with milk is that Crohn's disease is triggered, in 90 per cent of cases, by a bacteria found in milk, including pasteurised milk, and in water.

Foods which may contain milk products, and therefore lactose or milk proteins, include biscuits, bakery products, sausages, processed meats, chocolate, non-dairy creamers, protein powder drinks and creamy salad dressings. The ingredients listed on packaged foods may include casein, caseinate, lactose, sodium caseinate or whey, all of which are dairy derivatives.

Goat's and sheep's milk, and their products, have all got lactose in them and may still be troublesome for those with a lactose intolerance. However, they have different types of proteins, which means that if it is the protein aspect of cow's milk products which is causing discomfort, there is a possibility that goat's or sheep's milk products may be tolerated. For a full rundown on dairy alternatives see Healing with E.A.S.E., page 112.

CHAPTER SEVEN

Water, Water, Everywhere . . .

What is the second most important life-giving substance after air? What is the main ingredient in your body, accounting for around 70 per cent of your make-up? What is a universal solvent which keeps all the necessary molecules in your body in solution? What is a key ingredient in all enzyme reactions which run every aspect of your body's mechanisms, from keeping your heart beating, to allowing your kidneys to filter and your lungs to exchange gases? The answer is: water.

It is easy to take water for granted, after all, it is available at the turn of a tap, yet we need it for every function of our bodies. And one of the most important of these functions is the successful manufacture of digestive enzymes. Without regular replenishments we quickly become dehydrated and our health suffers. And yet one of the most common misconceptions is that when we are bloated, especially when we are retaining water in our body tissues, we do not need more water, because we have enough already. Nothing could be further from the truth. We need MORE. Nothing flushes out water faster than . . . water. One way of looking at it is to think of water retention as stagnant water in a reservoir which needs to be flushed out and replaced with healthy supplies. The standard way of getting rid of excess water retention is to use diuretics. These only relieve the symptoms and do not address the cause of the problem. It is like draining the reservoir, but not looking at the filtration system which, because it is faulty, allows the water to stagnate in the first place. The answer is to drink water. It has also been observed in studies that mild dehydration (of 5 per cent) increases the production of hydrogen gas and worsens flatulence.

Ideally, we need to drink two litres of water daily. It is normal for people to drink significant amounts of liquids, but frequently these tend to be dehydrating. And even worse, these dehydrating drinks also contribute chemical toxins which the body needs to be rid of. Coffee, cola and tea are the worst culprits in this regard. You can guarantee that, in Neanderthal times, cavemen and cavewomen did not put on the coffee pot when they were thirsty – they drank water.

We have evolved to drink water – anything else is a compromise. No other species on earth drinks anything other than water (unless in captivity). Of course there are other drinks which are not detrimental and, in fact do quite a lot of good, such as juices and herbal infusions, but we are meant to get a minimum amount of water daily, otherwise our health can suffer, leading to lethargy, stiff joints, aching muscles, headaches or disturbed digestion.

It can be quite difficult to convince long-term non-water-drinkers to create the new habit of drinking more water. The most common excuses are: 'I don't like the taste of it' (add some fresh juice to alter the flavour); 'I always forget' (set an alarm watch); 'I prefer hot drinks' (make hot water and lemon with a little honey); 'It makes me go to the bathroom too much in the night' (limit water intake after 6pm); 'I would find it hard to drink that much liquid' (measure out how much coffee and tea you drink, you will probably find that it comes to 1–2 litres daily); and so on . . .

In some people another possible cause of bloating is carbonated drinks or water. The carbon dioxide bubbles are not dispersed readily which can lead to discomfort.

WATER WITH MEALS

Many people feel that if they drink water with a meal it will dilute their digestive juices and lead to reduced digestive capability. However, fluids taken with meals actually stimulate optimal stomach acidity and trigger enzyme and bicarbonate secretion in the small intestine. Sipping water with a meal should help the digestive process. If you feel strongly that water with meals disrupts your digestion, the solution is to drink a glass or two of water, at room temperature, half an hour BEFORE a meal.

Part Three

A GUT FEELING

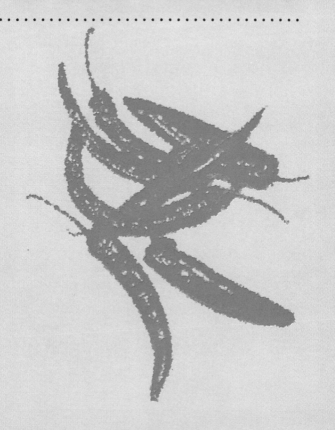

CHAPTER EIGHT

Introduction

Digestive problems account for a massive £150 million annual sales of over-the-counter medication in the UK and are the most commonly medicated conditions after the common cold. In addition, the National Health Service and Social Security between them foot a £1,600 million bill for digestive problems alone. Indigestion, ulcers, constipation, IBS (irritable bowel syndrome), colitis and the like plague our nation.

Compromised digestion is at the root of most bloating problems, and this can have a direct, or an indirect, effect. The direct effect is pretty obvious with food sensitivities and gas build-up being problems. But the indirect effect is also a big player in the bloating stakes, with water retention resulting from toxic metabolites from a poorly functioning digestive tract, and compromised liver health leading to hormone disruption.

We have around six metres of small intestines shaped like a coiled snake, and one and a half metres of large intestines or bowels. The total absorption area of the digestive tract is around the size of a tennis court and, during a lifetime, the human gut will handle around 65 tonnes of food and drink – equivalent to the weight of a dozen elephants.

For a healthy diet to translate into improved health the digestive tract has to be working efficiently. Let's look at what is involved in healthy and efficient digestion.

Digestion starts in the head. It even has a name – cephalic digestion (from the Greek word for head). If you are relaxed and content when you prepare your meal, you will already be salivating and secreting hydrochloric acid and enzymes in anticipation of your meal. If, on the other hand, you are anxious or under stress you may find that you are the type of person who is unable to secrete enough stomach acid or enzymes.

Stress shuts down the digestive tract, and the stress hormone adrenaline, which is designed to ready us for the primitive response of 'fight or flight', causes the supply of blood to shunt away from the digestive tract towards the skeletal muscles ready for 'action'. In the absence of action, the digestive tract remains with a reduced blood supply which limits digestion. The other important stress hormone, cortisol, inhibits repair of the tissues lining the digestive tract, which also reduces its effectiveness.

Addressing excessive stress is an important part of digestive health as it is commonly linked to intestinal hurry, IBS and ulcers. We are used to thinking of the stomach as the seat of the emotions and we have numerous expressions which reflect this, for example 'the collywobbles', 'butterflies', and the title of this chapter, 'a gut feeling'. Calm emotions are really the bedrock of good digestion.

CHAPTER NINE

The Mouth

This is the section of the digestive tract which gives us the most pleasure, where food and drink first enter the body and where we experience the flavours and textures of foods. You may well think that your mouth is just the part of the digestive tract where you shovel in food, and that the rest of 'the tube' is where the really important action happens. The mouth, however, actually has a critical role to play in the process of eliminating bloating and should never be underestimated. An astoundingly large section of the reflex control-centre of the brain is used to manage the lips, tongue and jaw, because the mouth is such an intricate and sensitive organ involved in taste, touch, smell, speech, digestion and breathing.

CHEWING FOOD

In our fast-paced world, where we eat without thinking, perhaps at our desk, in front of the TV or at a sandwich bar, it is not unusual to simply break up our food five or six times with our teeth before swallowing. Just enough effort is exerted to make the food swallowable. Often people will have sore gums which prohibits careful chewing, and healthy gums and teeth are important for the whole process of digestion.

One of the key contributors to bloating is undigested food putrefying and fermenting in the gut. If we do not chew our food properly we are not increasing its surface area enough to allow digestive enzymes to do an efficient job. The more digestive juices have to work at breaking up large chunks of food in our stomachs, the less effective they are and the greater the risk of bloating.

While there are some digestive enzymes in the mouth, food does not really stay in the mouth long enough for them to make a serious impact. The relationship of the mouth to enzyme production is an important, but not obvious, one. Signals received by the mouth forewarn the rest of the digestive tract about which foods are coming down it, and therefore which enzymes it needs to start producing in readiness. This stimulus is reduced if food does not stay in the mouth long enough for the feed-back mechanism to work properly.

An important message therefore is to chew your food properly and to eat in a relaxed environment. These steps will provide a useful start to reducing bloating.

TASTE SENSATION

Our tongue is the organ of taste, with areas of taste buds to sense bitter, sour, sweet and salt flavours. When taking action against bloating it is a good idea to develop a liking for the first two, bitter and sour, rather than sweet and salt. The reason for this is that an excessive amount of both sugary and salty foods is linked to bloating problems. We will discuss sugar in all its forms extensively in this book and it is sufficient to note here that sugar acts as food for unfriendly, gas-producing, bowel bacteria and is a major cause of bloating problems. If you are going to satisfy a sweet tooth, it is best to do so with fruits or other natural sources of sweetness as described in **Healing with E.A.S.E.**, page 119.

Salt is one of the major causes of water retention, which is a bloating of tissues referred to as oedema. You will be aware of how well salt retains water if you tip a little table salt into a plate and drip some water around it. It soaks it up immediately. The same thing happens in your body and in many cases salt also contributes to high blood pressure.

The food processing industry has made a fortune out of our addiction to sweet and salty foods. The reason that we have taste buds which are geared up to these two taste sensations is that they are, historically, important for our survival. During the course of our evolution the chances were that if we ate something sweet, such as a fruit, it was not going to poison us. Salt is necessary *in small quantities* for our survival, as it bears the essential mineral sodium. But we have not yet evolved beyond these basic survival taste mechanisms whereas the food processing industry has changed beyond all recognition in the last 50 years. With their eye on the profit line, the food manufacturers cynically add huge quantities of highly addictive sugar and salt to our foods as flavour enhancers and preservatives. At least 80 per cent of the 50 kg, or more, of sugar we eat annually, and the 9 g of salt we eat daily comes from packaged foods, and not from the sugar bowl or the salt cellar.

An absolute maximum of 6 g of salt daily would cut problems such as cardiovascular disease by about a third. To reduce salt levels, you need to dramatically cut down on packaged foods and use salt-free or low-salt products whenever possible. A bowl of cornflakes, for example, will give you 0.75 g of salt and a slice of bread will deliver 0.5 g.

An excessive amount of salt is often just a habit which needs to be addressed over time, but it can also sometimes be a sign of zinc deficiency. A daily supplement of zinc for two or three months may help the transition to a low-salt diet. The best source of added salt is milled seaweed flakes, which are available from health food shops – these give essential trace minerals alongside sodium. You can also exercise your cooking skills by becoming more familiar with strong tasting, and health giving, herbs and spices.

HUNGER SIGNALS

Another link between the mouth and bloating is hunger. There is definitely such a thing as 'mouth hunger' rather than 'stomach hunger'. True hunger is felt in the stomach, but the kind of hunger that says, 'well I just feel like a little bit of . . .', is probably mouth hunger, and is the type most likely to lead to overeating. An excess of food should not be underestimated as a cause of bloating. It could be triggered just by the sheer volume of food sitting in the stomach or intestines, or it could be that there are insufficient digestive enzymes and the overload is affecting the digestive process. So, the next time you think you'll have something 'just to round off the meal' consider eating it at a separate sitting, for instance as a snack.

Another mistaken signal of mouth hunger is thirst. We frequently mistake thirst signals as hunger signals, and drinking a glass of water is the real solution. See **Water, Water, Everywhere . . .**, page 31.

BAD BREATH

Before we leave the mouth and head it is worth mentioning the subject of bad breath. This can be a symptom of bloating. Assuming that mouth hygiene is good, excessively strong bad breath is usually a sign of maldigestion. The fumes literally float up the oesophagus from the stomach into the mouth. A furred up tongue can be caused by excess toxins being eliminated, and this is frequently experienced when a person goes on a detoxification diet and begins to throw off accumulated, stored toxins.

CHAPTER TEN

The Stomach

The stomach, when empty, is about the size of a clenched fist, but is capable of expanding to accommodate 1.5 litres. The cells lining the stomach produce hydrochloric acid (HCl) which has a pH of around 2.0 – acidic enough to burn a hole in your carpet! But the stomach is clever and has a coating of mucus which protects it from self-assault.

The reason the stomach is such an acidic environment is that this is where protein digestion begins. Pouring acid on proteins is the first step in breaking them down. The proteins are curled up tightly and HCl begins to unwind them ready for digestion.

Protein digesting enzymes are produced in an inactive form, otherwise they would digest the lining of the digestive tract. They are only activated if sufficient HCl is present. Proteins are found in most foods, and it is the protein component of grains, the gluten, which causes many digestive problems, especially bloating.

HCl also stimulates the pancreas to secrete fat and starch digesting enzymes, and the gall bladder to release bile for fat digestion. This feature makes it important for digestion of all types of food. Sufficient acidity is needed to trigger cholecys-tokinin, a gut hormone, which tells us when our hunger is satisfied. Insufficient HCl can mean the message 'I am full' does not get through, prompting us to eat more. Finally, and of great importance, the acidity in the stomach is the means by which many 'foes' – viruses, bacteria, yeasts and parasites – are killed off, keeping us in good health.

So this humble acid is vital for effective digestion. You may think that all this seems fine because, as is widely believed, many people suffer from excess stomach acidity. Yet many more people have low stomach acidity than they do high.

LOW ACIDITY

Confusingly, the symptoms of low stomach acidity and excessive acidity are virtually the same, which has led to a lot of misdiagnosis in the past.

Rather than high acidity being the culprit in cases of stomach ulcers, these are frequently the result of low acidity allowing the 'ulcer bug' *Helicobacter pylori* to proliferate in the stomach. As with other bacteria, a good level of stomach acidity is necessary to kill them off. When this does not happen, *H. pylori* manages to get a foothold and ulcerates the stomach and duodenal lining.

Even more confusingly, antacid medication which is prescribed for high acidity seems to temporarily resolve low acidity problems, with the result that using antacids as a means to confirm high acidity has also led to misdiagnosis.

Symptoms of low stomach acidity can include excessive burping after a meal, bad breath, indigestion, heartburn, a feeling that food is slow to move out of the stomach, bloating, a sense of fullness after eating, flatulence and constipation or diarrhoea. The symptoms are likely to be more pronounced after eating a protein based meal.

The factors which can be involved in low production of HCl include a poor diet, stress, overeating and bolting food, low thyroid function, a genetic predisposition, anaemia, asthma, chronic yeast infection with candida and advancing years. HCl production seems to decline markedly in the general population from the age of 40–50. This may be related to low zinc levels as it is the mineral which is most important for HCl production.

Health Department figures show that 31 per cent of men and women get less than the recommended dietary intake for zinc, see **Healing with E.A.S.E.**, page 144 for information about improving stomach acidity levels.

CHAPTER ELEVEN

The Small Intestines

. . . .

You may have the best possible diet and take handfuls of good quality supplements, but if you do not digest and absorb well, it is likely that your health will be below par. As the bulk of digestion and absorption takes place in the small intestines its health is fundamental to our overall health.

The lining of the small intestines is deeply folded with millions of tiny finger-like projections called villi which have the effect of increasing the surface area for absorption. If they are damaged then malabsorption and malnutrition can take place. Because there are different areas of absorption for specific nutrients, it is possible for malabsorption of particular nutrients to happen if a particular area of the villi is compromised, for instance if there is local inflammation. This may explain why a person can be found to have a particular mineral deficiency despite taking supplements for a period of time.

DIGESTIVE ENZYMES

Digestive enzymes are produced by the pancreas and poured into the small intestines, as well as being produced by the lining of the small intestines themselves. Many people have reduced pancreatic effectiveness which can contribute to a wide variety of health problems, one of the most obvious signs of which is bloating.

Production of digestive enzymes is in tune with the typical diet eaten by that person. When someone habitually eats meals which are high in protein (e.g. meat, cheese, eggs, soya), their pancreas will secrete up to seven times the usual amount of protein digesting enzymes. If, however, a person's diet is high in starches (e.g. bread, rice, pasta, potatoes), their pancreas will produce up to ten times more starch splitting enzymes. The major conclusion that can be drawn from this is that any significant adjustments to diet need to be made slowly, rather than overnight, otherwise the digestive capability of the enzymes will be out of synch with the new diet being eaten.

TRANSIT TIME

The time that food spends in the digestive tract dictates how effectively it is absorbed, and whether it has the time to cause mischief while it is there. If food is going through too fast, nutrients cannot be absorbed effectively. If the food in the digestive tract hangs around for too long, toxins are too readily absorbed. The digestive tract is the ideal place for food to putrefy as it is so warm and if transit time is poor then this leads to stagnation and decay. If the tube is sluggish, or obstructed, so that wind is not expelled speedily, this is felt as trapped gas and gives a sensation of bloating. Some of these gases can also become reabsorbed into the bloodstream and contribute to headaches and other feelings of unease. Fibre is the main dietary factor that affects transit time. It is a 'regulator' – speeding up slow moving matter, and slowing down matter that is going through too fast. If you are constipated, then the use of laxatives is detrimental in the long run. While they may solve the immediate crisis it is easy to become dependent on them and they result in a poorly functioning bowel.

Food ideally takes around 8–18 hours to pass through the whole system, but in reality it more commonly takes 24–36 hours. One way to check transit time is to do a sweetcorn test. Swallow a tablespoon of tinned, or cooked frozen sweetcorn, without chewing it. The kernels will not be digested if it is not chewed as the fibrous coating is too tough. You can then see very clearly when the kernels are passed out in the stools. Take the sweetcorn with your evening meal. If it is passed out in much less than 8 hours that is probably too quick. If takes more than 36 hours to appear that is too slow. As your digestion improves you can re-run the test and chart changes in the transit time. Some people are sensitive to sweetcorn and it can make bloating worse, however as the kernels are not chewed this test does not usually present a problem.

CHAPTER TWELVE

Balanced Bowels

In those with a healthy digestive tract only a small amount of waste products are eliminated in the faeces, and if there are significant amounts of protein or other undigested and unabsorbed food this is a sign of a malfunctioning digestive tract. A popular misconception is that we eliminate the waste products of our diet in our stools. The major routes of excretion of waste products, which have been metabolised in the body, is through the urine, the skin and the lungs. Faecal matter consists of bacteria that is housed in the digestive tract, indigestible fibre from plant foods, water and other substances (e.g. haemoglobin and bile salts). Bowel movements should be bulky and easy to pass, not small, like rabbit pellets, and difficult to pass. A saying I am fond of is, 'Big stools, small hospitals'.

The bacteria in our guts are so numerous that they weigh around 1–2 kg, and one-third to two-thirds of the main mass of stool weight consists of gut bacteria, most of which are still alive when they are passed out in stools.

THE GOOD, AND THE BAD, GUYS

Most of the bacteria in the small intestines are aerobic, and thrive in oxygen, while those in our bowels are anaerobic, and thrive without oxygen. Anaerobic conditions favour bad, or putrefactive, bacteria. The three main types of beneficial bacteria are:

- *Bifidobacteria*

- *Lactobacillus acidophilus*
- *Lactobacillus bulgaricus*

The word 'bifido' means good and, as the name implies, *Bifidobacteria* are the main family of good bacteria. *Lactobacteria* get their name from 'lacto', meaning milk, because they produce lactic acid, which was first known as the agent generated during the souring of milk to make products such as yoghurt. *Lactobacteria* are present on grass and on vegetables and grains, and the fact that cows eat grass accounts for the presence of *Lactobacteria* in their milk.

We have bacteria everywhere in us, and on us, in vast quantities. One millilitre of saliva alone can contain anything between 10,000 and 1 billion micro-organisms. Beneficial bacteria are actually in the minority and are outweighed by harmless and 'bad' bacteria. In the worst cases of disrupted digestion, the beneficial bacteria can be so low in number as to be virtually undetectable. In the healthy digestive tract the beneficial bacteria keep the activities of the bad bacteria in check. Not only does their physical presence prevent the bad bacteria from proliferating, they also produce mild antibiotics against their room-mates. It is a case of survival of the fittest.

The main functions of the good bacteria include:

- The final digestion of proteins.
- Helping the digestion of lactose (milk sugar), by producing the lactase enzyme.
- Producing lactic acid, which keeps the bowels mildly acidic, is necessary for a healthy bowel and helps prevent bowel cancer.
- Killing off harmful organisms and making natural antibiotics to deter unfriendly bacteria. These help prevent food poisoning and diarrhoea.

- Manufacturing usable amounts of vitamin K, the blood clotting vitamin, and the B-vitamins B1, B2, B3, B6, B12 and folic acid.
- Producing butyric acid from dietary fibre, which feeds the cells of the digestive tract and in so doing keeps it healthy.
- Stimulating contraction of the walls of the bowels.

So important are the good bacteria to our immune systems that, in experiments, it was found that if animals were kept in a completely sterile environment from birth, and did not acquire any of the beneficial bacteria in their guts, they did not develop and thrive normally. In particular, they were immunologically crippled with poor development of digestive lymph tissue.

Part Four

WHAT CAN

GO WRONG

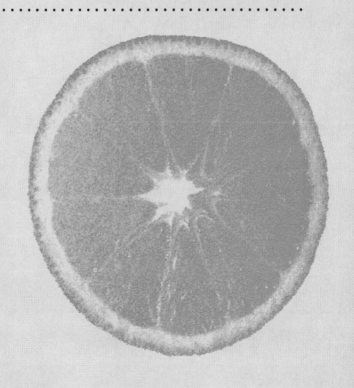

CHAPTER THIRTEEN

Introduction

The flow chart below shows the vicious circle that can occur. The starting place could be anywhere on the chart, but the most likely place is with inflammation. In this chapter we will follow the chart around in sequence to understand the dietary and lifestyle factors which are likely to contribute to the problem of bloating. Once we understand this then we can look at solutions.

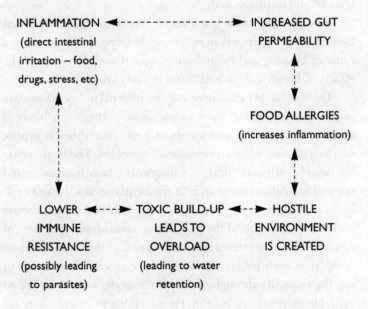

INFLAMMATION ◄------------------► INCREASED GUT
(direct intestinal   PERMEABILITY
irritation – food,
drugs, stress, etc)

                                                                    FOOD ALLERGIES
                                                                    (increases inflammation)

LOWER ◄---► TOXIC BUILD-UP ◄--► HOSTILE
IMMUNE   LEADS TO   ENVIRONMENT
RESISTANCE   OVERLOAD   IS CREATED
(possibly leading (leading to water
to parasites)   retention)

CHAPTER FOURTEEN

Inflammation

It easy to see inflammation on the surface of our skin. The smallest splinter can result in quite a lot of inflammation. People who are susceptible to acne, rashes and eczema all exhibit visible inflammation. Exposure to a substance which irritates, such as washing powder or insect bites, can lead to external inflammation that is visible. But when this inflammation takes place internally, not only can we not see it, but it is often ignored and misdiagnosed.

Inflammation of the gut lining is one of the most important factors to consider when rectifying bloating. It is not only a cause of bloating and related symptoms, it is also a result of the effects of bloating. A vicious spiral is easily created.

The indications that there may be internal inflammation are often non-specific and hard to recognise – tiredness, lowered immune resistance, bowel upsets. Chronic diarrhoea is usually due to irritation and inflammation of the colon. The term irritable bowel syndrome (IBS), is a diagnosis which is often meted out and is totally non-specific. It frequently means 'I don't really know what is wrong with you, but you obviously have some underlying irritation of the gut'. IBS accounts for 50 per cent of referrals to gastroenterologists and is one of the most common complaints seen by your doctor. I have mostly chosen not to use the term IBS throughout this book as the symptoms are so varied from person to person. The one thing you can be sure of, however, is that IBS, if you have been diagnosed with it, will involve inflammation somewhere along the digestive tract.

Inflammation can be caused by a number of things: food

allergies, bowel bacteria imbalance, medication, parasites, chronic stress, nutritional deficiencies. I discuss the first five throughout the book, so will focus here on deficiencies.

NUTRITIONAL DEFICIENCIES AND INFLAMMATION

Some nutrients are particularly important for keeping inflammation in check. It is not unusual for these to be deficient in the diet, or for them to be malabsorbed because of disturbed digestion. The key nutritional deficiencies, or imbalances, which can lead to excessive inflammation are:

Antioxidant nutrients

The main antioxidant nutrients are the vitamins A, beta-carotene, C and E, and the minerals selenium and zinc. There are many other antioxidants which we get from our diet, such as anthocyanidins in red and purple coloured berries and lycopene from tomatoes and pink grapefruit. The best sources of antioxidants are all fruits and vegetables, including legumes which are beans, peas and pulses.

The job of antioxidants, as the name implies, is to prevent oxidation damage to tissues. Oxidation damage happens because of the action of free radicals (a major source of which come from the oxygen we breath, and from the processes of meta-bolism and digestion). Free radicals are unstable electrons which, in an attempt to stabilise themselves, pinch electrons from our cells which damages those cells and the tissues they make up. A major cause and effect of free-radical damage is the inflammatory process. Antioxidants help by, in effect, sacrificing themselves. They give up electrons which would otherwise come from our cells. Therefore, the more antioxidants we obtain from fruits and vegetables in our diet, the less we sacrifice our own body tissues to this process. A minimum of five 80-g portions of fruit and vegetables daily is the figure to aim for, and more is better. As well as helping to suppress inflammation in the digestive tract, fruit and vegetables also contribute fibre which is so important for good digestive function. Occasionally, people bloat when they eat fruit, in which case they may be better off favouring vegetables until their digestion is sorted out.

Particular antioxidant nutrients, vitamins A and C, and the mineral zinc, are also vital for tissue repair. Once inflammation has set in, if there are insufficient building blocks (proteins and healthy fats) and vitamins then repair will be slowed down. For example, vitamin C is needed for the process of building collagen, the glue which sticks our skin and mucous membrane cells together and A, C and zinc are all necessary for repair to inflamed tissue.

B-Complex

This group of vitamins is important in maintaining an efficient immune system and low levels are linked to suppressed immune function. If the immune system is running below par, inflammation is more likely to get out of control. B-vitamins are also used for energy production in every cell, and for healthy cell replication, making them important in successful tissue repair. B-vitamins can be found in whole grains, leafy green vegetables, brewer's yeast, beans, pulses, dates, figs, molasses, egg yolks, shellfish and liver.

Healthy fats

These consist of two groups, omega-3 fats and omega-6 fats and include the essential fats. The richest sources of omega-3s are oily fish, such as mackerel, sardines, tuna, salmon, but they are also found in flax oil, linseeds, pumpkin seeds and walnuts and their oils. The richest sources of omega-6 fats are evening primrose oil, sunflower, sesame and safflower oil, and all nuts and seeds. Most vegetables also contain omega-6, though at low levels. To benefit from any of these sources, the oils must be cold-pressed, must not be stored for too long and must be kept refrigerated – if they aren't they go rancid. It is also helpful to have these fats in the correct balance, and there is a tendency in a Western diet to have too many of the omega-6 fats at the expense of omega-3s.

Both of these classes of fats have strong anti-inflammatory actions. They keep inflammation in check by countering the effects of a substance called arachadonic acid, which encourages inflammation, and is derived in the diet from animal fats such as red meat, butter, cream and full-cream milk.

Another critical function of the omega-3 and omega-6 fats is that they are used as building blocks for skin and mucous membrane repair. They are needed to fix the damage of the mucous membrane lining the digestive tract after inflammation has subsided.

If the diet favours too much red meat, or full-fat dairy produce at the expense of oily fish, nuts, seeds and vegetables, this can encourage a hyperinflammatory state in susceptible individuals. In practical terms, too much meat would be equivalent to more than one modest portion a day.

MUCUS

One of the signs that inflammation is rampant in the gut wall is the production of excessive and unhealthy mucus. The linings of our tube are described as mucous membranes, from the lining of the mouth all the way down to the rectum.

The mucus produced plays a necessary part in protecting the digestive tract and helping food to slip along it. Healthy mucus is clear and slippery. Unhealthy mucus is cloudy, thick, sticky and may be yellow in colour. Many people are susceptible to producing excessive, unhealthy mucus in reaction to specific foods, in particular cow's milk, dairy products, gluten grains, soya, sugar and red wine, although other foods may also cause it. Unhealthy mucus is also triggered by allergens such as pollen and house dust mites. The mucus formed from food or airborne allergens is apparent with stuffed-up noses, nasal drips, and phlegm. Unhealthy mucus can also coat significant portions of the digestive tract – it just isn't so immediately obvious.

Unhealthy mucus can contribute to the problem of bloating because it creates a thicker than normal barrier between the lining of the tract and partially digested carbohydrates. The final stage of carbohydrate digestion is governed by enzymes which are produced by the villi which form the lining of the tract. The remaining carbohydrates, the disaccharides or two-sugars, are unable to be broken down because of the thick mucus barrier, and so remain available to gut bacteria for a feeding frenzy. This can lead to gases building up and to bloating. A vicious cycle then follows because the response to substances that bacteria produce, and to yeasts, is to produce more mucus.

If stools have got mucus in them they will be less bulky than healthy stools, and because the faeces are 'sticky' they pass out of the bowels less easily than their healthy counterparts. The more mucus in a stool, the more sticky it will be and the longer it will take to pass, with possibly more straining. If it takes ten minutes to pass a stool, even if you go daily, this suggests that you are constipated.

CHAPTER FIFTEEN

Gut Permeability

The lining of our small intestines, when healthy, is designed to allow through only certain substances into the bloodstream. These substances are properly digested proteins, fats and starches and the vitamins and minerals they contain. These components are then used by the body for healthy growth, repair and functioning.

Absorption happens via a number of mechanisms through the cells themselves or at special junctions between the cells. The spaces between the cells are called tight-junctions which, as the name implies, are closely fitted together and do not normally allow unwanted substances to pass between them.

HELP – I'VE SPRUNG A LEAK!

Problems start when there is irritation or inflammation and the tight-junctions loosen up. This allows normally unabsorbable molecules to cross the barrier and be taken into the bloodstream. These molecules are then seen as foes and cause the body to mount an immune attack. If this is allowed to continue, the lining of the wall is increasingly damaged so that even larger molecules are allowed through, as well as bacteria and toxic molecules. This causes an even greater immune reaction, resulting in oxidation damage at the site of the 'battle', further damaging the lining of the gut wall.

This condition has been nicknamed 'leaky gut syndrome' and has been associated with a number of conditions, including bloating, food allergies, asthma, bronchitis, eczema, psoriasis, coeliac disease, Crohn's disease and rheumatoid arthritis.

The lining of the gut wall can also be disrupted by decreased, rather than increased, permeability. This condition is explained in greater detail in **Gluttons for Gluten**, page 24. The same set of measures are used to heal this problem as for increased permeability – avoid what is causing the disruption, and give the cells what they need to repair themselves. So, while the two conditions are different and lead to slightly different symptoms – though bloating is common to both of them – for treatment purposes the two conditions are the same.

CAUSES OF ALTERED GUT PERMEABILITY

What leads to altered gut permeability? There are many factors which can contribute to disruption of the functioning of the gut lining, and in most people they probably have a cumulative effect. Sometimes, as in the case of harsh medication such as chemotherapy, there is known and rapid disruption to gut functioning and this can lead to altered gut permeability in a few days.

Some people may have had gut permeability disruption since childhood. This can happen because they have been exposed to disturbing influences very early on, for example gluten grains at too young an age. It is possible, for instance, to develop coeliac disease in babyhood. A baby's gut lining is much more permeable than an adult's, and does not reach the same integrity as an adult's digestive tract lining until the child is around two years of age. Many of the foods which are disruptive, such as dairy products, gluten cereals, soya and citrus fruit are notable for being the first foods we introduce to children – meaning that we are risking setting up gut permeability problems from the outset.

The factors that are most likely to contribute to altered gut permeability in adulthood are:

- **Constant stress** – elevated stress levels, over long periods of time, lead to a number of changes which adversely affect the digestive tract's ability to repair itself. Increased cortisol (a stress hormone) is produced which slows down tissue repair, less immune factors are secreted by the digestive tract, the blood supply to the digestive tissues is diverted away, and peristalsis (the squeezing motion of the digestive tract) is interrupted.

- **Food allergies** – these are discussed in some detail in the next section and they are a major contributor to altered gut permeability.

- **Alcohol** – this is disruptive when drunk to excess, although excess means different things for different people, depending on liver size and functioning. Alcohol is metabolised through the liver and its toxic residues have to be broken down and eliminated or stored in the body. Alcohol can overload this system, and lead directly to damage to the intestinal lining.

- **Bacterial imbalance** – an overload of toxic by-products from 'unfriendly' bacteria can cause inflammation and damage to the gut wall. Bacterial imbalance also sets up an environment which can permit the opportunistic yeast, candida, to get a foothold and invade the gut wall.

- **Medication** – over-the-counter medication (OTC), particularly painkillers and anti-inflammatory medicines have a direct effect on the gut wall, which can be so bad that it leads to ulceration. It is best to limit OTC medication as much as possible and to talk to your doctor about limiting any prescribed medication, such as steroids. Do not stop or decrease any prescribed medication without talking to your GP first.

● **Chemicals** – occasionally people are sensitive to chemicals and find that they do not recover fully and feel really well until they eliminate much of their exposure. Chemicals which can cause sensitivity problems include household cleaners, detergents, room sprays, insect sprays, perfumes, agricultural sprays and swimming pool chemicals, although many other substances can also trigger a reaction. It is often the case that addressing other health issues, for instance food allergies, will increase a person's tolerance to environmental chemicals.

TESTS FOR GUT PERMEABILITY

While there are a number of tests available to establish gut permeability, the mannitol/lactulose test is the most widely accepted and accurate. This test, to establish if you have increased or decreased gut permeability, is a simple one which you can carry out at home. It is readily available via a nutritionally trained doctor or a qualified nutritionist. The test involves drinking a sweet tasting solution and then collecting urine for analysis.

The sweet solution consists of two sugars, mannitol and lactulose, which cannot be used or metabolised by the human body. Mannitol, a tiny molecule, is normally easily absorbed by the cells of the digestive tract in people with a healthy gut. Lactulose is a large molecule which is not readily absorbed. These are possible test results:

● Someone with a healthy gut wall should have a test result that shows mannitol has been completely absorbed and

lactulose absorbed at very low levels.
- If high levels of both mannitol and lactulose are found in the urine then this indicates increased gut permeability, or leaky gut.
- If low levels of both mannitol and lactulose are found in the urine then this indicates malabsorption of all nutrients.
- Low mannitol, with high lactulose levels is a possible indicator of coeliac disease, ulcerative colitis or Crohn's disease, and such a result needs to be followed up with confirmation by other testing, and by dietary exclusion.

HOW TO FIX IT

If there is disturbed functioning of the gut wall, either increased or decreased permeability, or inflammation, then the cells lining the gut wall need to be repaired in order to achieve a return to optimal health. The healing methods for both conditions are the same, because the natural approach is to offer the cells of the gut wall what they need to stabilise themselves and repair damage. If you offer them the correct conditions and nutrients, they will be able to repair both forms of malfunction.

The first course of action is to avoid foods, drinks, drugs and lifestyle habits which may be irritating the gut lining and causing inflammation which leads to increased permeability, or induces malabsorption. It is helpful to identify if there are any other conditions which might be contributing, such as candida or parasites.

Once the 'causes' have been eradicated certain nutrients can be taken, in therapeutic doses, which feed and help to repair the gut wall. It is interesting that, of all the cells in the body, the cells lining the gut wall do not principally feed from the bloodstream, but directly from the contents of the digestive tract. This means that the quality of the diet intimately affects digestive health. It also means that any therapeutic agents are able to have a very direct effect on healing the tissue. The substances do not have to circulate around the body to get to where they need to be targeted. There are a number of nutrients and specific formulations that can be helpful, and these are discussed in **Healing with E.A.S.E.**, page 153, and listed in **Appendix II**, page 186.

CHAPTER SIXTEEN

Food Allergies

The word allergy means aversion and has its roots in the Greek word *antipathes*. In orthodox medical circles, the term allergy is strictly applied to substances which cause an instant immune reaction in an individual. These immune reactions can be quite severe, resulting in hay fever, asthma, hives, rashes, vomiting, swelling of the breathing passages and, in the most severe cases, death. This sort of immune response is easily measured with a blood test looking for a type of reaction called an IgE antibody. Almost any substance or food can cause this reaction, but it is most likely to be found in airborne allergens, such as pollen and house-mite faeces, insect bites and stings, and detergents. The most common food culprits are peanuts, sesame seeds, egg whites, dairy products, soya, shellfish, fish, citrus fruit, and some highly coloured fruit such as cherries.

More recently, a group of food related problems have been acknowledged as the cause of a wide variety of health problems. Because they do not trigger the classical IgE reaction which can readily be tested for, their relevance has been the subject of debate amongst more orthodox physicians. To compound the confusion these reactions to foods have been grouped under the heading of allergies, when strictly speaking they should probably be grouped separately as sensitivities or intolerances. Internal inflammation as a result of a reaction to food has, in recent history, been hotly disputed by many specialists. We are currently seeing the renaming of conditions such as IBS as allergic colitis, suggesting that food is now viewed as a possible cause of irritation of the gut wall. To the lay person these differentiations are pretty irrelevant – if a food causes an unpleasant reaction, then they will have an aversion anyway.

The main distinguishing feature between IgE allergies and food sensitivities or intolerances is that the latter are reactions which can show symptoms anytime up to 72 hours after eating the food. This makes them difficult to diagnose. These reactions are also commonly linked to foods which are eaten very frequently.

One of the key symptoms of food sensitivities and intolerances is bloating. This can be caused by inflammation of the lining of the digestive tract, or due to wind as the foods are not broken down properly. They can also cause water retention, and exacerbated hormonal bloating. These resulting symptoms can be dramatic and alarming in some people. The types of food which are most likely to trigger food sensitivities or intolerances are covered in **Eat Your Food (Don't Let it Eat You!)**, page 11, and in **Healing with E.A.S.E.**, page 102.

PROTEINS CAN PUTREFY

Low stomach acid levels allow food to 'putrefy' as it sits undigested in the digestive tract, leading to many unpleasant symptoms. The results of putrefaction, as anyone knows, are unpleasant smells from the gases given off. If proteins are not digested sufficiently they can pass into the bloodstream and set up allergy or food intolerance reactions which can lead to inflammation and excessive water retention as the body tries to neutralise these foes. Because of these knock-on effects of low stomach acidity, it is very useful for anyone who suffers from bloating, wind, indigestion, bowel problems or food intolerances to establish if low acidity is a problem. The simplest way to do this is to take an HCl supplement with meals to see if it helps to relieve any of the symptoms, although you should not

take one if you have ulcers. It may also be useful to have a trial
period to see if food combining is helpful, by not overloading
the stomach with starches during protein digestion, see **Healing
with E.A.S.E.** pages 144 and 129 for a full rundown of both.

TESTS FOR FOOD ALLERGIES, SENSITIVITIES AND INTOLERANCES

There are a number of tests available to determine if particular
foods are likely to be a problem. These are the most popular:

RAST (Radioallergosorbent test)

This involves measuring the antibody response to suspected
food allergens. It is quite effective, but not foolproof, and does
not identify food intolerances.

Skin test

Involves pricking or scratching the skin and applying the suspect
substance, or injecting the substance under the skin. If a red
weal appears then the food is deemed to cause an allergic
reaction. Again, it is not foolproof, and can produce some false
positives. This is unsurprising as it is not a normal route for
allowing food into the body! Skin prick tests do not identify
food intolerances.

ELISA (Enzyme-linked immuno-sorbent assay)

This is a blood test which measures a different type of antibody,
the IgG antibody. This is a type of immune response which has a
'short-term' memory. A food can trigger an IgG response, but if
the food is avoided for six to eight weeks, the IgG response is

usually 'forgotten' by the immune system. The IgG response is not reprogrammed unless the food is eaten regularly for several consecutive days. The food can, theoretically, be reintroduced and, as long as it is not eaten more than one day in four or five, will not reprogramme a reaction. While the IgG reaction is often life-long, it can be controlled in the short term by this means. This test can have its uses, but it may not be totally accurate and the long list of foods reported with some of the ELISA test results can often lead to an unnecessarily restricted diet.

Cellular allergy test

A blood test which measures leukotrienes response to any foods. This is useful for true allergens as well as intolerances. While it can give mixed results, it may be a bit more reliable than the ELISA test.

SIgA

This is another component of the immune response located in the digestive tract. Increased levels of SIgA are produced when foods which irritate it are consumed. Testing for raised levels of SIgA can be useful in determining if there is inflammation of the digestive tract lining, however it is non-specific about which foods might be causing the trouble. There is a gliadin-SIgA which can identify if there is a problem with the gluten grains.

Elimination and reintroduction

This is the most reliable test, as long as it is carried out correctly. It is also the cheapest because you can do it at home on your own, but it requires motivation, discipline and careful organisation. This method is described fully in **Healing with E.A.S.E.**, page 110. It involves totally avoiding the suspect foods for two weeks, and then reintroducing them in a controlled fashion, one by one, on different days to ascertain which are the culprits. During this time a careful note should be kept of which symptoms disappear on avoidance, and which reappear on reintroduction.

Kinesiology

This is a system of uncovering imbalances by testing the response of muscles to certain influences. Kinesiology uses a mixture of chiropractic muscle information and Chinese energy, or meridian, flows. The therapy is used for a number of health issues, including structural/muscular and emotional problems. As far as food testing is concerned, the theory is that certain foods, to which the individual is sensitive or intolerant, will interfere with the energy flows in the body and, at one level or another, interfere with muscle function. Nobody knows how this system really works, but work it does in many cases. This therapy is very dependent on the practitioner being experienced. In the hands of a practitioner who knows what they are doing, it can be remarkably accurate, and yet in the hands of a novice it can be next to useless. Nevertheless the 'biofeedback' from accurate testing can be very motivating.

Other tests

There are other testing methods which are not particularly accurate and the results are difficult to replicate if required. These include pulse tests, hair and nail analysis, vega testing and dowsing.

CHAPTER SEVENTEEN

A Hostile Environment

. . . .

Potential lodgers and squatters – viruses, yeasts, fungi, parasites and harmful bacteria – are present in our food and environment and are ready to move in to our digestive tracts at the first opportunity.

When there is an imbalance of bacteria in the small intestines or in the bowels it is referred to as dysbiosis. Dysbiosis is the opposite of symbiosis, which means organisms working together for a common benefit. Dysbiosis means that a war is on. In your bowels. The term, dysbiosis, was first coined by Dr Eli Metchnikoff, who in 1908 won the Nobel Prize for his work on the bacteria *Lactobacilli* and their role in maintaining human health. He was also a colleague of Louis Pasteur, the father of the 'germ theory', and succeeded him as director of the prestigious Pasteur Institute in Paris.

Metchnikoff's work focused on the balance between the friendly bacteria which colonise our bowels, and the unfriendly bacteria which can move in and disrupt the internal environment. The unfriendly bacteria produce toxins which, he reasoned, led to ill-health by creating more work than the body was capable of dealing with.

A more user friendly term for dysbiosis is bacterial imbalance. Bacterial imbalance can reduce our ability to protect ourselves from disease-causing microbes, such as *Helicobacter pylori*, *Klebsiella*, *Salmonella*, *Citrobacter* and *Staphylococcus aureus*. It also leaves the door wide open for the yeast candida to invade the digestive tract from its normal home in the bowel. These little critters can lead to a wide range of symptoms, including bloating, flatulence, diarrhoea, cystitis and ulcers, as well as the more instant symptoms of food poisoning such as vomiting, bowel purging and fever.

CAUSES OF BACTERIAL IMBALANCE

Bacterial imbalance is usually the result of a number of conditions which, over time, lead to chronic overgrowth of 'bad' bacteria at the expense of 'good' bacteria. The most common lifestyle and dietary factors which influence this are:

- **Overuse of antibiotics** – Antibiotics are not selective and will kill off bacteria whether good or bad. Immediate relief of symptoms, as bad bacteria are eliminated, is often accompanied by a worsening of the symptoms, or the appearance of seemingly unrelated symptoms when the antibiotics are stopped. For instance, acne may be successfully treated initially, only to return more virulently at a later date. It is very common for people to experience bowel problems, including bloating, gas and loose stools, after several courses, or even just one course, of antibiotics. There is now, thankfully, a reluctance to overprescribe antibiotics and a move towards reserving them for when they are truly needed to treat virulent and dangerous bacterial infections. However, recent surveys have shown that, in the UK, antibiotics account for 12 per cent of all prescribed drugs in adults (27 per cent in children!) and that at any time one million people are taking antibiotics. You also need to be cautious about some supplements, as even natural antiseptic ones such as goldenseal and grapefruit seed extract can reduce the levels of beneficial bacteria if taken over a long period of time.

- **High levels of sugar, alcohol or refined carbohydrates in the diet** – Bacteria of all types feed on sugars and starches. This type of diet is like preparing a picnic for both good and bad bacteria, but mostly for the unfriendly bowel bacteria. They celebrate by producing lots of gas and toxins which can trigger inflammation of the gut wall and water retention – all of which are experienced as bloating.

- **High levels of stress** – High levels of stress alter the integrity of the mucous lining of the digestive tract and reduce the ability of beneficial bacteria to adhere to it.

- **Low stomach HCl levels** – These allow unfriendly bacteria to pass into the intestines. A normal level of HCl in the stomach would kill off many of the pathogenic bacteria.

- **Slow transit time of food through the intestinal tract** – This can encourage bacteria to be in the tract for longer than is desirable and the longer they are inside us, the longer they have the opportunity to colonise our bowels. In 24 hours just one E.coli bacterium will multiply sufficiently to produce around 5,000 bacteria.

- **Pharmaceutical drugs** – Long-term use of the contraceptive pill, steroids, aspirin or other NSAID (Non-Steroidal, Anti-Inflammatory Drugs) medication, encourages proliferation of the unfriendly bowel bacteria by changing the mucous lining of the intestines which support the bacteria. NSAIDs are also heavily implicated in problems of increased gut permeability.

TESTING THE 'ENVIRONMENT'

A very useful test for determining the environment of the digestive tract is the CDSA test – the Comprehensive Digestive Stool

Analysis. This is available through doctors trained in nutrition, and nutritional therapists. The laboratory technician can work out if sufficient digestive enzymes are being produced by checking whether food is properly digested or remains in the stool. They can measure immune reactions and inflammation by examining SIgA, mucus levels and the presence of any blood (though the presence of blood should always be a reason to visit your GP). They check the levels of certain bowel bacteria, both beneficial and putrefactive. The CDSA can also look for parasites in the stools, though this is often best accompanied by mucus swabs. It is common to team up the CDSA with a gut permeability test. The test is not cheap, but can be a mine of useful information. Of course, you do not need a test to get well, but this one can help to pinpoint the exact reasons for bloating and therefore shorten the treatment phase.

NATURAL ALTERNATIVES TO ANTIBIOTICS

Following the advice in this book should help create a healthy immune system and improved acidity in the stomach. These first lines of defence are the most important tools you have when faced with bacterial invaders. In order to avoid the need to use antibiotics unnecessarily, which are the drugs most likely to devastate the healthy bacterial colonies in the bowels, you may find it useful to bolster these natural defences with some natural antibiotic agents which do not have the same broad-spectrum effect, and in some cases selectively target unhealthy bacteria, while promoting healthy bacteria.

Garlic – the ultimate natural antibiotic.
Colloidal silver – a superb and multipurpose preparation.
Grapefruit seed extract – a potent antibiotic, though overuse
   can lead to disruption of healthy bacteria.

St John's wort – more usually thought of as an aid to beat mild depression, St John's wort has also been shown in trials to be an ally in the fight against the drug-resistant 'superbugs' found in hospitals.

Echinacea – this is not an antibiotic, but it supports the immune system response to bacterial invaders.

Oriental mushrooms – maitake, reishi and shitaki, support the immune response. Add three or four reconstituted dried, or fresh, mushrooms to your meals daily.

Digestive enzymes – if used early they can help to literally digest the early stages of a food poisoning type of bacterial invasion in the digestive tract.

CANDIDA

Candida is present in our bodies normally, but generally lies dormant and does not create a crisis. It is when candida is able to proliferate that it may cause problems. It is an opportunistic yeast which thrives when there is bacterial imbalance in the bowels. This type of yeast overgrowth causes thrush of the vagina and mouth, and sometimes the nailbeds or eyes. The usual culprit is *Candida albicans*, but there are other species as well. Candida exists in two different forms. There is the non-invasive, yeast-like version, then there is the invasive form which spreads in the same way that other yeasts and mushrooms do, by microscopic threads. These threads or 'roots' can infiltrate the membranes lining the digestive tract, making it more open to inflammation and leakiness of food molecules into the blood-stream. Candida can produce around 80 powerful toxic by-products, resulting in allergic-type reactions which lead to a wide variety of possible symptoms, including abdominal bloating, vaginal infections, cystitis, 'jock itch', fatigue, premen-strual syndrome, insomnia, mood swings, and sensitivities to perfumes, cigarettes, moulds, damp days, chemical odours and other environmental conditions.

Candida is most likely to occur in those with a history of repeat use of antibiotics, in long-term users of the contraceptive pill and steroid medications, and in those who follow high sugar or alcohol diets. Antibiotics have a limited effect on candida, so when the antibiotics diminish bacterial colonies, the candida is well placed to grow and fill the gaps left behind. Candida has tended to be over-diagnosed in the recent past as little was then known about increased gut permeability, which can cause similar symptoms, and which is, of course, a related problem. Treatment of presumed candida often worked as it probably had an indirect beneficial effect. It is now possible to give a more fine-tuned diagnosis and treatment of these different problems. Nevertheless, candida is a valid diagnosis for some people and treatment can bring remarkable relief of symptoms.

Testing for candida overgrowth is notoriously difficult and inefficient. With current testing procedures (blood, stool and swab), identifying whether candida is truly a part of the whole picture, or if the test results relate to different factors, can be a problem. Treatment includes eliminating the overgrowth of candida, healing the gut wall, supporting the immune system and restoring the balance of bacteria, see Healing with E.A.S.E., page 135.

CHAPTER EIGHTEEN

Toxic Overload

Inflammation, increased gut permeability, food allergies, sensitivities and intolerances, bowel bacteria imbalance, candida – either in isolation, or in combination – can all be part of a vicious cycle which, in turn, can lead to a build up of toxins.

They can overburden the body's detoxification systems and lead to toxins having to be stored in body tissues – resulting in bloating on a grand scale, or aches and pains in joints. An overburdened detoxification system can also mean that toxins cannot be dealt with efficiently, causing direct health problems such as headaches, migraines and asthma. The most obvious example of the latter is when we drink too much and get a hangover the next day. This is partly caused by dehydration, but a major contributor is an excess of the toxic alcohol metabolite, acetaldehyde.

Toxins are processed via the liver and it is there that they are neutralised and packaged for excretion. We excrete these principally via the urine and the skin, and to a lesser degree via the breath and the bowels. Some toxins are circulated in the blood and the lymph system, where they are neutralised by the immune system.

If circulation in the lymph is sluggish, which is most apparent when people are dehydrated, or if the liver is overloaded and cannot handle the sheer volume of matter to be processed, the toxins must be stored ready for the day when there is 'spare capacity' and they can be offloaded. This may also be the case with someone whose genetic make-up means their liver is less able to deal with toxins.

Toxins are stored in the liver, and in fat cells. The storage of toxins in the fat cells is probably a significant contributor to cellulite, a common female woe. In some people this is quite evidently related to particular foods which, when consumed, increase the girth of their thighs quite substantially within a few hours. When these foods are avoided this form of bloating does not happen.

The processing and storage of toxins by the liver is also a key player in female hormone balance and the effect on cyclical, monthly water retention and bloating that hormones have.

Signs of excess toxicity can be bad breath, a sour taste in the mouth, and unusually malodorous urine and sweat. Toxicity is also a contributor to unpleasant smelling faeces. In his book *The Colon Health Handbook*, Robert Gray tells the story of a yogi in India who passed 'perfumed-scented faeces' from his body. Gray initially thought this phenomenon was due to the yogi's special spiritual powers or was at the least a sign of high spiritual development! At a later date, however, he himself managed to duplicate this effect by switching, for a while, to a fruitarian (fruit-only) diet. If you want perfumed-scented stools, you now know what to do! I ought to say, however, that fasting does not suit everybody and can be too rigorous. I would not advocate it unless under supervision of a qualified health professional.

POTTY TRAINING

It is very important to the correct balance of bacteria in the bowels to make sure that you evacuate your bowels daily. Only around a third of adults open their bowels once a day, which is the minimum for healthy elimination. You can address this issue by ensuring that you have sufficient fibre in your diet, sufficient water intake and that food sensitivities are addressed (see the relevant sections in this book). If all of these measures do not work then you may want to consider these additional tips.

Most people are embarrassed to talk about their lavatory habits, but sometimes it is necessary to spell it out. We have been conditioned to think of defecating as impolite. No matter how relaxed we think we are, most of us will ignore the urge to go if we are in a public place. It is important to get into the habit of taking time to go to the loo every morning at least, and to not rush it. How you sit on the toilet can make a difference to successful bowel movement. We are designed to squat and not to sit. The squatting position brings different muscles into play which favour peristalsis, the squeezing motion of the digestive tract. You can simulate this by upturning a waste-paper basket and placing your feet on it while you sit on the loo. It works!

If you remain constipated, you may want to investigate if a course of colonics is appropriate, bearing in mind that colonics have also helped with innumerable, and intractable, cases of bloating. It is important to find a well-qualified practitioner who you feel you can trust, as this is an invasive procedure, and I strongly suggest that disposable nozzles are used, rather than sterilised equipment. It is also helpful if they use a *Bifidobacteria* or *Lactobacillus* implant with their colonic. Some therapists may also use herbs which encourage healthy bacterial growth. Colonics are not suitable for some people and you should discuss your full health history with the therapist.

CHAPTER NINETEEN

Are You Being Bugged?

In our hygienic, sanitised and deodorised society it is unpleasant to think that we may be carrying parasites around. And yet wherever there is an opportunity in the natural world, some little beastie is ready to move in and make a home. It is not difficult to catch parasites of one sort or another – from restaurants where there is questionable hygiene, from overseas where water may not be well purified, even from your children, who have been exposed at school or playgroups, or from your pets. For many people, parasites may do little harm and there are no discernible symptoms. If you find that your bloating symptoms are not alleviated by other measures, it is always wise to think about the possibility of a parasite infestation. Parasites can often cause bloating, along with other digestive symptoms, including some, but not necessarily all, of the following: gas, constipation, diarrhoea, abdominal cramps, allergies, unexplained weight loss, anal itching, IBS, anaemia, joint and muscle aches, immune problems and bloody stools (blood in your stools should always be checked by your doctor). Any symptoms you experience may not be consistent, as they can fluctuate during the life cycle of the parasite.

It is generally assumed that with our improved standard of living the problem of parasitic infection has been eliminated, but this is not the case. As late as the 1940s many families, especially farm families, would not only worm their animals periodically, they would also worm themselves. It was probably with a great sense of relief that this practice was abandoned as the concoctions used, such as sulphur and molasses, were pretty unpleasant. These days preparations come in encapsulated forms, which are easy to take.

If you do find that you have parasites, it is wise to have the whole family tested and treated. It is not unusual for carriers to be symptom-free, which means they can re-infect those with whom they live at close quarters.

TYPES OF PARASITES

There are many different types of parasite, but for our purposes they can be divided into visible and microscopic.

Visible parasites include pinworm (threadworm), hookworm, roundworm, whipworm, fluke and tapeworm. (Ringworm is not a parasitic worm, but a fungal infection.) Pinworms are easy to detect as they are like tiny, white wriggly worms that come out of the anus, and the most common symptom is anal itching at night. In children you can simply examine for them, but for yourself you may find it easier to apply a little sticky tape to the area, and then to examine it. You may need to do this a few times.

The microscopic parasites of the digestive tract that are most common in Western countries include *Giardia intestinalis* (or *lamblia*), *Cryptosporidium parvum*, *Entomoeba coli*, *Entomoeba histolyca*, *Dientomeba fragilis*, *Blastocystis hominis* and *Endolimax nana*. We are surrounded by sources of parasites. For instance, cats are a source of *Toxoplasma gondii*, which can be dangerous for developing babies in the womb, and there are also sexually transmitted parasites such as *Trichomonas vaginalis*. Protozoa have a variety of different life cycles. The most advanced forms have cysts which protect them from damage when being transferred from host to host – this makes them very tough and difficult to destroy.

Some strains of parasite burrow into the tissues, such as the wall of the digestive tract, making them quite hard to eradicate. As with most health conditions, many people are able to keep parasite infestations under control, but when their immune or digestive health is compromised, or if they are in a vulnerable group such as the very young or elderly, symptoms become apparent.

TESTING FOR PARASITES

Random stool samples will be accurate about 80 per cent of the time. For some parasites, such as giardia, which live higher up the digestive tract, it is necessary to take special oral laxatives to flush them out, and this is called a stool purge test. As some parasites burrow into the mucous membranes lining the digestive tract, it is best in some instances to have a swab taken which removes some of the mucus. The mucus is often a better indicator of parasitic infestation than the stools. The most accurate screening for parasites uses all three methods: random stool test, stool purge test and rectal swab. If your doctor does not do these tests, a nutritionally trained doctor can organise them for you, see **Resources**, page 195. Parasites can also be looked for, and found in, blood, urine and sputum – but these are appropriate for parasitic infections other than digestive ones, such as malaria or toxoplasmosis.

AVOIDING PARASITES

In the chapter **Healing with E.A.S.E.**, page 161, various options are given to help eliminate parasites, however avoiding them in the first place is one positive step which can be taken:

Water quality Cysts of the two most common water-borne parasites can withstand chlorination at the levels used to

disinfect water (0.2–4.0 mg per litre). The only way to
guarantee that drinking water is free of cysts is to filter, or
even better distil, your water. Filters need to be one-
micron filters, or reverse osmosis filters.

Wash fruit and vegetables Parasitic cysts can be found on
inadequately washed produce, and organic produce can
often be a greater source of these cysts as animal fertilisers
are used in preference to chemical ones. Organic produce
is to be preferred over inorganic produce for a number of
health reasons, such as reducing exposure to chemicals,
however it is a good idea to wash it carefully. Water
vegetation, such as watercress, bamboo shoots and water
chestnuts, as well as fish, are a source of flukes.

Soak fresh fruit and vegetables in a bowl of water with
one tablespoon of vinegar for 15 minutes to remove and
destroy parasites and cysts, then rinse them. Cutting boards,
knives and cooking utensils should be thoroughly cleaned.

Cook meat and fish thoroughly Beef and pork, if undercooked, can be sources of tapeworms, and the roundworm
Tichinella. Raw fish, for example in sushi, gravlax, pickled
herrings and cold smoked salmon can be a source of
tapeworm, and undercooked fish has also been a source of
anisakid worm.

Wash your hands After handling babies' nappies, working in
the garden or handling animals, wash your hands thoroughly,
and use a nailbrush as parasites can lodge under the nails.

De-worm your pets Keeping pets healthy is the best way of
ensuring that they do not contaminate your family.

Part Five

IDENTIFY

THE PROBLEM

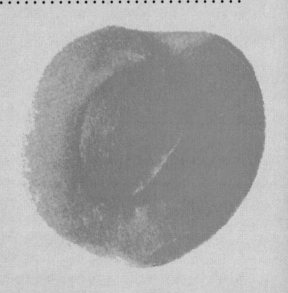

CHAPTER TWENTY

Your Digestive Health Profile

Now that we have examined the whys and wherefores, it is helpful to focus attention on your personal health history and what might be triggering the bloating you are experiencing. Finding the likely contributing factors is the first step on the road to eliminating the problem. Once you have decided what is involved, you can move on to the next chapter **Healing with E.A.S.E.**, page 95, and, while following the programme in sequence, focus specifically on the aspects which are relevant to you.

The following checklists will help you to identify your personal profile. At the end of each section add up the total number of points you have scored.

I. IS FOOD ALLERGY OR INTOLERANCE CONTRIBUTING TO YOUR BLOATING?

	TICK	SCORE
● Do you begin the day with a flat stomach with bloating developing during the day?		
Sometimes		2
Frequently		4
● Do you have fluctuating symptoms which seem to come and go		2
● Do you have a lot of trapped wind or flatulence on a regular basis?		4
● Do you suffer from water retention and weight fluctuations?		4

	TICK	SCORE
Do you experience loose stools or diarrhoea regularly?		4
Do you suffer from constipation?		2
Do you experience inexplicable fatigue during the day?		I
Do you have regular bouts of any one of the following symptoms: headaches, 'dry' nose, skin problems, eczema, excessive nasal mucus, hay fever, asthma, frequent infections?		2
Do you have inexplicable aching joints or rheumatoid arthritis?		2
Do you get periodic dark rings or puffiness around the eyes, not related to lack of sleep?		2

TOTAL SCORE: ....

2. COULD YOU HAVE LOW STOMACH ACIDITY?

	TICK	SCORE
Do you have bad breath from 'fumes' rising from your stomach?		2
Do you suffer from frequent burping?		I
Do you have a feeling of fullness for an extended period after protein based meals (e.g. meat, fish, dairy products, eggs, tofu)?		2
Do you tend to be constipated?		2
Do you suffer from unpleasant smelling flatulence?		2
Do you have any known food allergies?		I
Do you have signs of osteoporosis indicating poor mineral absorption?		2
Do you regularly use antacid medication?		2

TICK SCORE

● Have you been diagnosed with stomach ulcers? 2

TOTAL SCORE: ....

(The last two questions could relate to low stomach acidity resulting in infection with the bacteria *Helicobacter pylori*, or could be related to high stomach acidity.)

3. SIGNS OF INCOMPLETE DIGESTION AND POSSIBLE LOW LEVELS OF DIGESTIVE ENZYMES

TICK SCORE

● Do you have indigestion between 1–3 hours after
   eating? 2
● Do you suffer from trapped wind or from flatulence? 2
● Do you have any known food allergies or
   intolerances, or a score of 8 or more for
   checklist 1? 4
● Do you have a history of constipation or diarrhoea
   (especially alternating)? 2
● Are undigested food particles visible in your stools? 4
● Is there mucus in your stools (either visible mucus,
   or stools have a sticky consistency, or are poorly
   formed)? 2
● Do you have foul smelling stools? 1
● Do you have difficulty gaining weight? (should be
   checked by your doctor if this persists) 1

TOTAL SCORE: ....

4. IS INCREASED GUT PERMEABILITY AN ISSUE?

	TICK	SCORE
● Do you experience abdominal bloating or pain?		2
● Do you have a known food allergy or intolerance, or a score of 8 or more for checklist 1?		4
● Do you drink alcohol more than three times a week? ..		2
● Do you take aspirin or other pain relieving or anti-inflammatory drugs on a regular basis?		4
● Have you fasted for an extended period of time in the past, either intentionally, or unintentionally (e.g. because of anorexia or during illness)?		2
● Do you have a history of regular antibiotic usage (three or more times in a year, or one course for two months or more?		2
● Do you have inexplicable aching joints or rheumatoid arthritis?		2
● Do you have mucus or blood in the stools? (blood in stools should always be checked by your GP)		4
● Do you have ulcerative colitis, Crohn's disease or coeliac disease?		4

TOTAL SCORE: ....

5. DO YOU HAVE TOO LITTLE FIBRE IN THE DIET?

	TICK	SCORE
● Do you eat mostly white bread, rice and pasta, refined breakfast cereals, and have a high proportion of packaged and convenience foods in your diet, such as chips, crisps, pastries and biscuits?		4
● Are you constipated on a regular basis? (Constipation means having days when you do not pass stools or passing stools daily but having to sit on the lavatory		

TICK SCORE

for an extended period of time or strain or if the
stools are small and not bulky) 4

● Do you have loose stools or diarrhoea on a regular
basis? 4

● Have you had appendicitis, haemorrhoids, colitis or
diverticulitis, and not made changes to your diet? 4

● Have you had breast, prostate or bowel cancer, and
not made changes to your diet? 4

TOTAL SCORE: ....

6. COULD YOUR BOWEL BACTERIA BE OUT OF BALANCE?

TICK SCORE

● Do you have frequent flatulence, or trapped wind,
accompanying your bloating? 4

● Do you have a high meat or other animal protein
based diet? 2

● Did you score 8 or more in checklist 5, indicating
a low-fibre intake? 4

● Do you have frequent constipation, loose stools, or
diarrhoea? 4

● Do you have foul smelling stools? 2

● Do you have a history of frequent antibiotic usage
(three or more times in a year, or one course for
two months or more? 4

TOTAL SCORE: ....

7. SIGNS AND HISTORY WHICH MIGHT INDICATE A CANDIDA OVERGROWTH

TICK SCORE

- Do you have a known food allergy or intolerance or did you have a score of 8 or more for checklist 1?... 1
- Do you crave sugary foods, alcoholic drinks or bread? 2
- Do you experience regular bouts of vaginal irritation, anal itching, ringworm or 'jock itch', or do you get fungal infections of the nails or athlete's foot? 4
- Do you have a history of repeated antibiotic usage? (three or more times in a year, or one course for two months or more) 4
- Have you used the contraceptive pill for more than two years? 2
- Have you taken cortisone drugs for more than two weeks? 2
- Have you been pregnant two or more times? 2
- Do you experience inexplicable fatigue throughout the day? 1
- Are your symptoms worse on damp, muggy days, in smoky atmospheres, in mouldy places or when exposed to perfumes, insecticides or other chemicals? 2

TOTAL SCORE: ....

8. SIGNS THAT YOU MAY HAVE PARASITES

TICK SCORE

- Have you been to any developing countries? 2
- Have you been overseas (anywhere) and experienced digestive illness during your visit or within a month of returning? 4
- Have you ever drunk water from lakes or rivers

	TICK	SCORE
without first boiling or filtering it, while camping or hiking?		4
● Do you regularly eat unpealed, unwashed fruits, vegetables or salads?		2
● Do you frequently eat out in restaurants, especially ethnic, vegetarian, fast food or steak houses?		2
● Do you prefer meat or fish which is raw, or cooked rare or medium-rare?		2
● Do you use the same cutting board for meat as you do for vegetables?		2
● Do you frequently handle animals which may not have been wormed?		2
● Do you experience anal irritation?		2
● Is blood visible in your stools? (this must always be checked by your GP)		1
● Have you had an inexplicable loss of weight? (this should be discussed with your doctor)		2
● Are threadworms visible in stools or on anus		4
● Bloating and other symptoms, such as loose stools, do not clear up despite addressing other possible causes such as gut permeability or food allergies		2

TOTAL SCORE: ....

If your total score for any one checklist is four or more then suspect that the question raised may be a problem for you. If your score is over eight then the chances are high that you need to address this problem.

When deciding on your course of action for treatment it is best to read the whole book first. Then go to the next chapter, **Healing with E.A.S.E.**, and apply the treatment information sequentially in the order in which it appears, completing one phase before you go on to the next. You will probably only need to concern yourself with the sections which have been highlighted by completing these checklists.

The checklists are not intended as an alternative to seeking advice from your doctor, which you must do if any symptom persists and is a cause of concern to you.

Part Six

HEALING
WITH E.A.S.E.

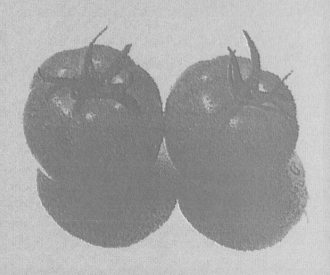

CHAPTER TWENTY-ONE

Introduction

We've looked at the various symptoms which might be expressed under the collective term of 'bloating'. We've looked at what might be the food related or physical reasons for such bloating. We've also looked at how to identify which are the most likely causes for you, based on your symptoms. Now for the really important part – how to banish bloating.

We need to promote effective digestion, starting with the mouth and continuing along the whole length of the intestines, ensuring correct nutrient absorption and bacterial balance along the way until, finally, there is healthy elimination.

The steps to take, in sequence, have been broken down into four steps with a programme called E.A.S.E. This programme owes much to the work of Dr Jeffrey Bland, a highly respected clinical nutritionist, in the state of Washington, USA. Here is a summary of the programme:

1. ELIMINATE THE CAUSE

This could involve identifying and eliminating foods which are causing sensitivities or allergic reactions, foods which encourage inflammation of the digestive tract, foods which fight with each other, or dealing with a possible candida overgrowth.

2. AID DIGESTION

Here we look at giving your digestive tract a chance to digest food efficiently by looking at when and how you eat, the possibility of using digestive enzymes if they are deficient, and other digestive aids.

3. SOLVE THE DAMAGE

A digestive system which has been under continued assault by foods which do not agree with it, toxic by-products of bacterial overgrowth, or possibly candida, will probably have sustained some damage to its basic fabric. Much can be done to encourage healing of the digestive tract and, if it is done successfully, there is less chance that the problems will recur.

4. ESTABLISH A FRIENDLY ENVIRONMENT

The final step is to create the right environment for continued digestive and hormonal health. By adding beneficial components to the diet, such as fibre and good bacteria, we can make sure that the lodgers in our digestive tracts are those which respect the property, clean up their mess and leave nice flowers for their host – not the type who create mayhem!

How much of the programme do I have to follow?
. . . .

This is a hard question to answer as it largely depends on what your particular problems are. Ideally, it is best to go through each section methodically, in sequence, to work out which ones are relevant to you. For instance, it may be appropriate to cut out a food to which you are sensitive, but it may be irrelevant to consider parasites. Or the reverse may be true. Taking each step at a time avoids clouding the issues and wondering which measure is really the effective one. It also means that you do not spend a fortune on supplements at any one time. Many of the benefits are felt at the front end of the Healing with E.A.S.E.

programme, and once your get further along you need only make fairly small adjustments and improvements here and there.

How long will it take?

The immediate rewards of making changes to your diet can be fairly swift, but to achieve lasting relief from bloating and other symptoms, perseverance may be required – it is best to think of these as positive changes for life. As already suggested, it is not sufficient to suddenly switch to a healthy diet and expect all to be well overnight. Years of disruption to the digestive tract can take a little while to resolve.

The more meticulously you stick to the advice, the more rapid the resolution is likely to be. You may find that you get significant relief within two to four weeks from implementing the first step – 'Eliminate the Cause'. And you may be tempted to stop there, happy with the results. However, to allow you to return to a 'normal' life, dietarily speaking, it will probably be necessary to follow through with the other three steps in order to avoid a backlash if you resume some of your old ways. It all depends on your tenacity.

You may want to work with a nutritionist and run laboratory tests to understand what is going on internally, measuring the production of digestive enzymes, the permeability of the gut wall and the populations of the bacteria in the bowels, so that you are able to be certain what changes are happening and in which time frame. However, this is only necessary if you are one of those people like to see what is going on in 'black and white'.

It may get worse before it gets better

The symptoms of bloating usually get better quite quickly if you address foods which may be causing or contributing to it. The exception to this is if, unwittingly, you begin to eat larger quantities of foods which you do not normally eat, and to which you have an adverse reaction. If this is the case, more sleuth work is needed to identify which might be the offending foods. Typically, what will happen is that wheat is eliminated from the diet, but then more oats or rye based foods are eaten. These may turn out to be foods which also trigger bloating and other reactions. If so, they will also need to be avoided at the same time.

It is not uncommon for symptoms associated with detoxification to increase during the early phase of eliminating foods from the diet. You may find that you experience headaches, a metallic taste in the mouth, cloudy or strong smelling urine or skin eruptions for a few days. This is a sign that the body now has an opportunity to throw off accumulated toxins. It should not go on for more than a week – in very rare cases it may go on for a bit longer, but this is unusual. Very occasionally, some people can feel quite unwell, which is a sign that they are detoxifying too quickly. This is not common where just a few foods are being avoided and is more likely to happen with a more rigorous diet, such as the Stone Age Diet.

Do I need to take all the supplements listed?

No. The preparations which are discussed are those which are the most tried and tested and usually offer good results. Many supplement companies have combined preparations with a number of the nutrients and herbs contained in one dose. The information in the following sections will help you to read the labels and to understand what is in these preparations. You may also find that one substance does not suit you, and the list provides other options to try. Wherever possible it is important to make sure that the substance is coming from the diet. So, for instance, when garlic or extract of berries is suggested, you can buy the supplements, but it is a better long-term strategy to ensure that you increase levels of these foods in your diet. If you are totally adverse to supplements, or cannot afford them, then you do not need to take them at all, though there is no doubt that they can speed up recovery and help to deal with more intractable problems.

CHAPTER TWENTY-TWO

E – Eliminate the Cause

The place to start, when banishing bloating, is to eliminate any foods from the diet which may be contributing to the problem. In the majority of people, this step alone will bring significant, if not total, relief. These foods are likely to be causing an allergic reaction, or sensitivity problem, and are probably encouraging inflammation in the digestive tract. Another possible foe which may need to be eliminated is an overgrowth of the yeast candida. Both are discussed in this chapter.

Which plan will work for you?

I have already discussed a number of foods that are likely to be a cause of bloating, and we will review which ones these are. However, first of all it is worth spending a little time talking about how to approach an elimination diet.

There are several ways to go about this. Many books talk about the one answer to all health problems. They sell books on the basis that they have found THE solution and that theirs is the best way forward for everyone. But as a consultant nutritionist I have discovered one absolute truth – THERE IS NO ONE DIET FOR EVERYONE. The reasons for this are:

- People have different physical constitutions.
- People have different lifestyles and eating habits which need to accommodate different eating plans.

— Not everyone is motivated in the same way, and we all have
   differing mind-sets and differing levels of addiction to
   certain foods. How profoundly we are affected by our
   health can have a dramatic effect on our adherence to
   various regimes.

Practically speaking, I have found that there are four regimes, or
ways of eating, that are successful at eliminating bloating and
related problems, and you will probably find that you prefer the
sound of one option over the other. They are as follows.

● **THE AVOIDANCE AND REINTRODUCTION PLAN**
  This is the most straightforward approach and the one
  which will suit most people. It involves identifying the
  food or foods, or drinks for that matter, which might be
  contributing to your bloating. The advantage of this
  approach is that you only tackle a small number of foods at
  the same time and, because there are so many substitutes
  for commonly disruptive foods, there is no need to feel
  deprived or to risk being on too restricted a diet. The
  disadvantage of this plan is that, because it is does not take
  a blanket approach to foods, it is possible that some foods
  which are contributing to the problem may be missed out.
  This plan will probably work for 50 per cent of people.

● **THE STONE AGE DIET**
  This is a much more radical approach that involves eating
  in a way that our hunter-gatherer ancestors would have
  done, avoiding all modern-day food processing innovations.
  Because it is stringent, it is best employed by people who
  have tried and failed with a number of other approaches
  before. It is a diet favoured by doctors working as
  allergists. The advantages are that the rules are very

straightforward – only a very basic number and type of foods are eaten. Foods which have been avoided are eventually introduced, though processed foods are not permitted. The disadvantage of this approach is that it is difficult to implement unless you are happy to prepare most of your food from scratch, as you cannot rely on shop-bought food. It can also play havoc with your social life. Care must also be taken to avoid falling into the trap of eating too restricted a diet. Most people will benefit from the Stone Age Diet, though most will find that one of the other three approaches will work just as well for them.

● AVOIDING FOODS WHICH FIGHT

This option is based on the food combining diet and is a simplified version without all the exceptions to the rules – which are sometimes hard to remember. The basic principle is that protein foods and starches are digested in different parts of the digestive tract and if they are eaten together they 'fight' and impair digestion. Around 25 per cent of people benefit from this approach and once you get the hang of the diet it is quite easy to implement – mostly you just have to learn to say no to the bread and potatoes, or to the meat, fish and cheese. The disadvantages are that it pretty much precludes eating desserts, and you have to be very selective about convenience foods such as sandwiches.

● THE ANTI-CANDIDA PROGRAMME

This is really just for people who have identified that they have a problem with candida, and it will work for around 25 per cent of people. If you do not have candida it will do you no harm to go on this diet, and it may even do you quite a lot of good, but will not necessarily resolve your bloating problem as you may still be eating foods to which you are sensitive. If, however, you do have candida, it is the quickest way to resolve your problems. It is possible that alongside this diet you may need to avoid foods that you have identified you are sensitive to. This diet is also dependent upon taking a number of supplements. All the other regimes can be followed with or without supplements, but there is no doubt that this diet is more effective if you follow the advice about supplements and tackle the candida problem from all angles.

Preparing yourself

Read the full account of the four plans before making up your mind which one is best for you. And if one does not work for you, then you can always give the others a go. In making your choice of system remember that you need to take your lifestyle into account. Think about possible pitfalls:

— Do you need to take lunch into work?
— When do you eat your main meal?
— Do you allow sufficient food preparation time?
— How active is your social life?
— What about the constraints and needs of your family?
— How much willpower do you have?
— What are your particular food addictions?
— Have you planned for enough substitutes?

Any exclusion diet needs a degree of willpower – or 'won't power' (I won't eat this . . .). Starting when you are not pre-pared, mentally or physically, is likely to lead to inconsistent results. Some people are lucky and can just flick a switch in their brain and say 'from this moment on I will not eat this'. But most people, mere mortals, need to prepare the ground.

Pick a time when you can devote some time to yourself and when your list of commitments is not too long. Warn your family and friends that this is the way it is going to be for a while. Clear the shelves of foods which will tempt you. Make a special trip to the supermarket to buy lots of substitutes, and while you are at it devote extra time to checking out new products and the positioning of products you need on the supermarket shelves. If you have a family who will be eating foods you need to avoid, clear out one cupboard and one fridge shelf just for yourself. Make sure the freezer is stocked up with single portions of foods you enjoy. If you are keeping gluten-free bread in the freezer, make sure you slice it before freezing so that you can just pop one slice in the toaster when you need to. Make life easy for yourself, not more difficult.

The most important tip of all is to include a lot of foods that you really enjoy, as the last thing you should feel is deprived. If you have to do without your favourite toast for breakfast (when most of us are at our weakest) buy lots of luscious mangoes, or stock the fridge full of your favourite spreads to put on rice cakes. Pre-plan for the times that might trip you up. If you keep at it, you will find that new habits replace old, and the foods you reach for on the shelf will be the ones that do not give you trouble.

When you have decided which plan to follow, make a list of all your favourite foods and look up tantalising recipes. For a suggested shopping list of foods that are free of the most likely problem-causing ingredients, see Appendix III. Most of the products are available at health food shops, and a gratifying number are now available at large supermarkets. You may also find that your local ethnic shop has many interesting alternative foods – be adventurous!

Eating at work or on the run

Adherence to most eating plans falters when lives are busy. If you find yourself eating on the run much of the time, or having to send out for lunch to the local convenience store or sandwich shop, you will find it helpful to plan ahead. Spend some time visiting the available shops and figuring out what you can eat which will fit in with your chosen plan. This type of preparation can make all the difference. When you are at your most hectic, it is not the time to make the difficult decision between a burger or a salad – you know which one will probably win! Here are some ideas:

- Your sandwich shop may well do jacket potatoes with a variety of fillings. If they do not carry a filling that suits you (say tuna, coleslaw or baked beans) ask them to keep a little stock for you – most small shop owners can be very co-operative. They may also have a soup of the day which will suit you, and many of them will now do salad boxes.

- The rise of sandwich sections in supermarkets and departments stores is an indication of how many people avail themselves of this type of fast food. Many will have salad boxes in the chilled section. You can also visit their deli section and find a wide range of cold cuts and Mediterranean-style dips. A quick visit to their fruit and vegetable section will yield some fruit to snack on and pre-cut crudités.

- If you have a takeaway ethnic restaurant near you, you may occasionally want to treat yourself to a vegetable curry or to stir-fried prawns and vegetables.

- Keep a selection of snacks in your desk drawer for those moments when hunger strikes – oatcakes, rye crackers, rice cakes, fresh nuts, fresh seeds, dried fruit.

- If you have a fridge at work stock up with some things at the beginning of each week – yoghurt, dips, cold cuts.
- If you have the facility to heat up food at work try some of the very good fresh soups that are available, or you could even heat up a portion from your previous evening meal.

Food addictions

The cruellest truth of diet manipulation is that we tend to be addicted to the foods that are most likely to be bad for us. It is pretty obvious why this happens with, for example, alcohol. But why does this happen with other foods?

Many foods, especially refined starches, trigger blood sugar 'highs'. To avoid going into a subsequent blood sugar low we may crave some more sugar or biscuits or cake. A more successful way of managing this is to eat a piece of fruit, an oatcake or to have a plain yoghurt. Other foods will create an adrenaline rush which makes us feel instantly good. This is most likely to be the case with foods and drinks to which we are 'addicted', such as coffee, sugar, wheat or cheese. What happens is that these foods initiate an emergency response which triggers adrenaline and, in truth, we are really addicted to the adrenaline fix. Other foods, in particular gluten from wheat and casein protein from milk, seem to produce substances which are very similar to mood-altering morphine-like chemicals in the brain. Knowing how addictive mind-altering substances are, this supports the idea that we can be addicted to certain foods. The real problem is that all three mechanisms seem to be associated with some foods, making it that much more difficult to kick your habit.

Keeping a food diary

It can be very useful to keep a food diary for a week or two to work out which foods are likely to be related to your bloating problems. Write down everything you eat and drink, record the times when you consumed them, and how you felt during the meal (whether you were in a hurry, or relaxed, or tense, and so on). You also need to make a careful note of the time and the intensity of any adverse symptoms which you experience. Over the course of a week or so, you should be able to identify which foods, drinks or circumstances are likely to trigger attacks. You can use the table in Appendix I to help you. You may find this exercise requires discipline, but it really is a tried and tested way of finding out what is likely to be a problem.

PLAN 1: AVOIDANCE AND REINTRODUCTION

To work out if you have a food allergy, sensitivity or intolerance, you must first decide what foods may be leading to your symptom of bloating. Having read this book thus far, you will, by now, have a clear idea of the most likely culprits, but you must also suspect all foods and drinks which you take regularly, especially if you feel very attached to them. For instance, it is common for coffee, tea, alcohol, potatoes, bananas – which are often consumed very regularly – to be a cause of bloating, in addition to the more likely suspects of wheat, dairy products, soya and sugar.

Eighty per cent of the food we eat comes from only ten foods. This occurs because of our personal food choices, but is aggravated by the ingredients which are added to packaged foods. For instance, you may not consciously be a soya eater, but it is added to a vast array of packaged foods. Wheat and dairy derivatives, which are cheap and plentiful, are also used to bulk out a vast number of packaged foods.

This limits the nutritional value we get from our diet, and means that repetition of exposure to some foods leads to an overburdening of our capacity to handle them. The two main problem-causing foods are dairy products and wheat, closely followed by other grains, soya, oranges and potatoes. Excessive sugar, alcohol, coffee and tea also cause reactions, but not usually via the route of food sensitivity – they deplete the body of nutrients, increase the stress reaction, play havoc with blood sugar, and contribute to bowel bacteria imbalance.

Working out what causes individual digestive problems can be a bit of a hit-and-miss affair. If you find that the most likely foods do not resolve your problems totally there are other foods and drinks that can be considered. These are some other frequent problem foods: fatty foods, spicy foods, fizzy drinks, chocolate, peanuts, corn, citrus fruit, fruit juice, tomatoes, peppers, cruciferous vegetables (cabbage, broccoli, Brussels sprouts, cauliflower, kale, etc), the onion family (onions, leeks, garlic, etc).

Frequently, however, these are not the main cause of the problems, and are secondary to the more likely candidates such as wheat and dairy products. Indeed, some of these foods, the cruciferous and onion families, can help to resolve digestive health in the majority of the population. Not being able to tolerate foods such as onions and cabbage may well be a sign of a severely disturbed digestion, rather than the foods themselves being bad for the person and, while they may need to be avoided initially, there should be no concern about seeing if they can be reintroduced once digestion has been improved.

How to avoid and reintroduce
. . . .

Avoiding all your suspect foods at the same time is the best approach. If you do not follow this tactic, you may find that the reaction to one food is masking those of another food. Make a list of all your suspect foods:

1. _____   2. _____

3. _____   4. _____

5. _____   6. _____

Avoid all the above foods, strictly, for 14 days, remembering to check the ingredients list of any shop bought or packaged foods you eat. It is important, however, not to have an overly restricted diet, and for a list of alternatives to wheat, gluten grains, dairy products, sugar and caffeinated drinks see the following sections.

During the 14-day avoidance period, keep a list of any symptoms which improve, stay the same, or get worse.

After the 14-day exclusion period, reintroduce the foods ONE AT A TIME every second day. For example, you might reintroduce yoghurt, then goat's cheese, then a yellow cheese, then milk. Reintroduce a quantity which would be considered a normal portion, for instance 75 g of cheese or a glass of milk. When the food is reintroduced make a note of any symptoms which return, within a couple of hours, or even within the next two days. Once you have tested the food, continue to avoid it, whether it has produced any symptoms or not, until you have tested all the other foods you are aiming to reintroduce.

The reintroduction is just as important as the avoidance period. You may find that you get an acute return of the symptoms which have abated, or you may find that you get different symptoms, for instance mouth ulcers or loose stools. Or you may not have any symptoms returning at all.

When you have identified the foods which are related to

your bloating, or other health problems, you will need to carry on avoiding them for a further two months. After this period you can reintroduce them into your diet to see if they have any effect. Some people will be able to tolerate the reintroduced foods, while others will find that there is a recurrence of problems. If you are able to tolerate the food, you will probably find that, if you abuse it, you will be back to square one. However, a rotation diet, where the food is eaten every fifth day, usually means that the food can be eaten without too much trouble. An example rotation plan for grains and dairy products is given later in this chapter.

If, after the avoidance and reintroduction tests, you have not found a link between specific foods and your bloating it could be that they are not involved. This does not mean abandoning the plan overall because you will probably find that addressing other areas (e.g. bacterial balance, parasites or fibre intake) is your answer. It could also be that you have not succeeded in finding the culprits, and that you need to investigate further with, for instance, The Stone Age Diet, page 121. There is only one instance when avoidance and reintroduction can be harmful and that is with a hypersensitive individual with bad asthma. In this case there is a small risk that reintroducing a problem food can trigger a severe asthma attack. If you are severely asthmatic talk to your doctor about this.

Alternatives to dairy

Gone are the days when a dairy intolerance meant that a diet had to be restricted. There are many excellent dairy substitutes commercially available based on soya, rice, oats, coconut and almonds. All of these are lactose free and are usually well tolerated by people who have dairy intolerances. Of all the substitutes, soya is the most likely to create further intolerance problems because it is a member of the bean, or legume, family and is sometimes poorly digested, see **Beanz Meanz Wind**, page 173. You can experiment with the following:

Rice milk A sweet tasting milk which is usually well tolerated but can sometimes cause fermentation problems in very susceptible people.

Soya milk A very versatile alternative which is ideal for cooking. Sometimes causes problems in sensitive people.

Soya yoghurt The type with live bacteria is the best to use. The fruit flavoured soya yoghurts usually have sugar added.

Soya cheese Best used for grilling on top of dishes.

Tofu A tasteless soya bean curd block which comes in firm or soft textures, and which takes on the taste of the dish to which it is added. Used for stir frys, marinated for kebabs or sandwiches, cubed into soups or fruit salads. It is ideal to use instead of milk in 'milk' shakes.

Oat milk Usually very well tolerated and ideal for cooking. May occasionally cause bloating in very susceptible people.

Coconut milk This creamy milk is best if diluted by at least half and makes a delicious substitute for cream in dessert dishes.

Almond milk This can also be made with cashews, and hazelnuts. It is not commercially available, but easy to make. Blanch one cup of almonds by pouring boiling water over them and letting them stand for five minutes. Pop them out of their skins. Put them in a blender with 1/2 cup of water and blend on a high speed. Add more water until you achieve the consistency you want – cream or milk – then filter through a fine sieve. The resultant milk will keep in the fridge for 48 hours. If you have too much sediment left in the sieve then you have not blended the mixture for a sufficiently long time.

Goat's milk/Sheep's milk Goat's and sheep's milk, yoghurt
and cheeses can often be tolerated by people with a cow's
milk allergy. Exclude them during an avoidance period for
dairy products, but when you reintroduce them you
will probably find that they are well tolerated.

Gluten grains

The main gluten grain which causes problems is wheat (found
in bread, pasta, pastries, biscuits, cakes, etc). Many people
avoiding wheat find that they can happily eat the other gluten
containing grains and products such as oats, rye, barley, spelt,
couscous and sprouted wheat, though they are all best avoided
during the initial two-week avoidance phase.

Oats Porridge oats, oatcakes, oat flapjacks and oat biscuits.
You can find many oat-based products, but check the label
to make sure that they do not contain wheat. Oats can be
used as a crunchy topping for sweet and savoury baked
pies. Whole rolled oats can easily be made into a flour in
your food processor on high speed.

Rye Rye was the grain used in England in the Middle Ages,
and it is still used in Eastern Europe today to make a firm
textured bread. It is difficult, but not impossible, to find
100 per cent rye bread in bakeries and supermarkets in the
UK. However, it is often combined with wheat flour and,
generally speaking, the lighter coloured and textured the
bread is, the more wheat flour it has in it. Dark, flat
German rye bread, and pumpernickel bread, is readily
available and has a slightly sour, but pleasing, taste. A
hundred per cent rye crackers are also widely available,
just check the label to make sure that wheat is excluded.

Rye can cross-react with wheat antibodies and some wheat intolerant people will find it needs to be avoided as well.

Barley This is a much under-used grain, which is usually only put in winter stews. It can be cooked and served in the same way as rice, as a side dish, added to salads or as a base for many dishes.

Spelt This is an old strain of wheat, which many people who need to avoid modern wheat find they can tolerate. It can be used in the same way as normal wheat flour for baking. Occasionally you can find 100 per cent spelt flour bread in speciality shops. Must be avoided during the avoidance phase.

Tricale A cross between wheat and rye, which is sometimes tolerated. It is available as flakes and flour. Must be avoided during the avoidance phase.

Couscous This is also wheat, but again a different type which may be tolerated by those avoiding modern wheats. It cooks very quickly by steaming, making it virtually a fast food.

Sprouted wheat Bread made from sprouted wheat grains is available from health food shops and it has a delicious chewy texture. Make sure the product has no ordinary wheat flour in it. Because the grain has been sprouted it loses some of its allergenic potential for some people. Must be avoided during the avoidance phase.

Alternatives to gluten

Bread and pasta provide a starchy base to a meal which is satisfying. Finding other starchy standbys is not at all difficult, however, though some people find that starches are a problem across the board and may need to be even more radical in their food choices. Here are some of the alternatives if you find that you can eat starches.

Rice A very familiar grain, which is available in many different strains, though brown rice is always a better source of fibre and nutrients. If cooking brown rice seems to take too long, you can make a bigger batch, as it keeps well in the fridge for three days, or you can freeze portion sizes. Rice cakes, rice flour, rice pasta and Chinese rice crackers, the latter being a delicious snack option, are all useful store cupboard stand-bys.

Corn Available as maize meal (polenta), cornflour (corn-starch), sweetcorn, popcorn and corn pasta, corn is the most common allergy causing grain in the US, but it seems to be well tolerated if people are not overexposed to it. There are many corn products available such as tacos and nachos, as well as recipes for corn bread and cakes based on maize.

Quinoa An Andean 'grain' which is not a grain at all. It does, however, cook like a grain and can be used as a substitute for rice, or be mixed in with rice. It makes a good base for more filling salads when served cold, or can be used as an alternative to couscous.

Buckwheat Despite its name, this is not related to wheat at all. Buckwheat noodles are readily available and are the basis for Japanese udon dishes. Buckwheat pasta and flour are also easy to find. The flour can be made into blinis – flat, bready pancakes which are useful alternatives to bread – and recipes using it can be found in many cookbooks. Freeze them, interleaved with baking parchment, and then pop them in the toaster individually and add sweet or savoury toppings.

Millet Often thought of as bird food, millet is a very nutritious grain which can be bought in flakes and made into porridge or muesli or cooked as a grain and added to many dishes and salads.

Potato A useful starchy base to a meal if you are avoiding grains. Baked potatoes are the most nutritious, and if you are roasting or steaming them, leave the skin on for its nutrients and fibre. Potato flour can be made into potato cakes, using another, non-gluten flour alongside it.

Sweet potato Another useful root vegetable, which has even more fibre in it than potato. It can be cooked in all the various ways that potato can. You can also use yams in the same way.

Legumes Beans of all descriptions make a filling base to many meals, including soups and salads.

Chestnuts Chestnut flour can be used as a thickening agent or added to other flours to change the texture/taste.

Sago Made from the pith of palm and used for puddings.

Tapioca Harvested from the cassava plant, it is available as hard round grains or flour, which can be used as a thickening agent or for puddings.

Gram Gram flour, made from chickpeas, is readily available from Indian, or similar, shops and many Indian recipes use it. Lentil flour is also available.

Rotation plan

When you reintroduce offending foods, you may find that a rotation plan can reduce the chance of a sensitivity being triggered again. Also, if you have elected to cut out wheat, in order to avoid oats becoming a problem, eat them every fourth day. This is not as hard as it sounds and some people find it a lot easier to say 'This is a rice day', or a 'corn day', or a 'buckwheat day', during which they stick to these alternatives. A rotation plan for someone who is avoiding gluten grains and cow's milk products, and who does not mind cooking, could look like this.

Potato and Goat's Milk Day

Breakfast Soaked dried fruit with goat's milk yoghurt and ground seeds.

Lunch Baked potato, stuffed with hummus spiced with chilli and finely sliced red peppers. Large mixed salad. Fruit.

Evening Chicken breast roasted with marjoram, garlic and olive oil, served with very lightly sautéed onion, celery and mushroom, steamed potatoes and finely chopped mint. Fruit.

Quinoa and Buckwheat Day

Breakfast Egg, mushrooms and tomato. Fruit juice.

Lunch Buckwheat pasta salad, with tahini dressing. Include peppers, tomatoes, spring onions, fennel, radish and black olives (or any other vegetables or salads). If eating this at work, take in a portion of cooked buckwheat pasta and stir it in to the (shop-bought) salad at the last moment. Fruit.

Evening Stir-fried vegetables with seafood, served with quinoa. Fruit.

Rice and Sheep's Milk Day

Breakfast Rice puffs, rice milk, sheep's yoghurt and chopped fruit.

Lunch Salad Niçoise (green salad with runner beans, tuna, olives and anchovies), served with an olive oil and lemon dressing. Fruit.

Evening Vegetable curry (include broccoli, carrots, cauliflower and onion), served with brown rice. Fruit.

Millet and Sweet Potato Day

Breakfast Millet porridge, topped with stewed apple with cinnamon and ground seeds.

Lunch Thick soup (lentil, or leek and sweet potato, or thick spicy vegetable). Fruit.

Evening Baked salmon, served with Mediterranean vegetables (roasted garlic, aubergine, peppers and courgettes) and sweet potato. Fruit.

If you find a menu such as this too daunting because you do not have the time or inclination to cook, you can still follow a similar plan using more convenience foods. On your rice day, for instance, you could have rice puffs for breakfast, rice crackers for snacks, a takeaway soup or salad for lunch, and a rice based takeaway in the evening. On a corn day you could have corn-flakes for breakfast, low fat cornchips for snacks, a takeaway soup or salad for lunch, and corn pasta (available from health food shops) with bought-in tomato and herb sauce in the evening. It really is quite easy to make your own plan, as long as you invest the planning time initially.

Satisfying a sweet tooth

One of the more difficult aspects of cutting out, or cutting back, starches and other carbohydrates from the diet – especially for those with a sweet tooth – is avoiding desserts and other sweet foods. With a little practice and planning it is possible to enjoy some delicious options as most people can tolerate a little honey and a few nuts and dried fruits. This means that cakes, muffins and flapjacks can be made using almond or soya flour, in the case of severe carbohydrate intolerance, and rice and buckwheat flour, for those intolerant to gluten grains. Recommended cookery books can be found in the **Resources** section, page198.

Fruits can be made into coulis by blending soft fruit in a processor to make a delicious fruit sauce. I find that just mashing a banana releases sufficient sweetness to add to many dishes, sweet or savoury, and gives an interesting and sweet taste. Dried fruit can also be puréed in a blender, with a little water to make a very sweet sauce. A hundred per cent fruit jams are now available in most supermarkets and health food shops, which are delicious and indistinguishable from the sugar-laden version. I would avoid buying the diabetic, and sugar-free, versions as they will rely on sorbitol or artificial sweeteners for their taste. These do nothing to help to retrain a sweet tooth, and they are laden with substances which are difficult for the body to process.

You can also try a type of sugar called FOS (short for fructo-oligo-saccharides), as you may find that this takes the edge off the need for something sweet, see **Fab Fibre**, page 166. It can be added to drinks, cereals and desserts. When added to yoghurt, it gives it a much creamier and firmer texture. You can also add FOS to baked dishes, replacing some of the sugar, an added benefit being that FOS seems to be very good at adding moisture to baked foods. Putting in too much can increase bloating or overstimulate the bowels, however, as can any unexpectedly high quantity of fibre. It takes around 40 g of FOS to induce loose bowels (around four tablespoons).

Coffee and Tea

Many people find that they cannot have a bowel movement without their morning coffee. This is a reasonable indication that coffee is an irritant to their digestive tract and bowels. Amongst coffee's other crimes is that it reduces the uptake of nutrients from the food we eat, imbalances blood sugar levels, taxes the adrenal/stress response and loads the liver with toxins which have to be eliminated. It is also a highly addictive substance. Coffee can contribute to bloating problems and is best avoided.

There are many alternatives to coffee available, including different blends of chicory, barley, acorn and dandelion root, as well as fruit, herb and Red Bush teas. Sometimes the barley drinks can be a problem for those with a grain intolerance, and some of the drinks have quite a bit of lactose in them, which can be a problem for some. However, if you pick carefully you can find a number of different options, one of which will probably suit you.

These substitutes will not provide the temporary caffeine 'lift' of real coffee and tea, but if you shift your thinking to that of having a nice tasting hot drink, they can be very satisfying. Other alternatives are to squeeze some juice and top it up with boiling water, or to add boiling water to a slice of lemon with a little honey. Sometimes it is just the action of switching on the kettle that is important. Some herbal and fruit teas have more 'bite' than others – for instance lemon and ginger tea or mint tea. Cooled fruit teas make very refreshing drinks in the summertime. Normal tea is unlikely to have an effect on bloating, but in the interest of general health it is best to restrict yourself to three or four cups of weak tea a day, or to use decaffeinated tea.

PLAN 2: THE STONE AGE DIET

Our anatomically-identical forebears have only been around for between 40–80,000 years. That is not a very long time in relation to the total evolutionary scale. Our immediate ancestors were hunter-gatherers, and they did not go round the supermarket with their shopping trolleys. They expended the majority of their energy in seeking out food, water, safety and shelter. Food gathering was a major activity and diets consisted of whatever could be hunted, fished or scavenged, and a wide variety of plant foods was eaten, including leaves, stems, roots, fruits and seeds.

A few isolated communities are still living on a hunter-gatherer Stone Age Diet in South America and Africa and none of these groups show significant, or indeed any, incidence of the Western digestive complaints which plague our culture. They do not have bloating, ulcers, appendicitis, constipation, diarrhoea, IBS, colitis, Crohn's disease, coeliac disease, or colon cancer.

What they do get, automatically, by eating in this way is in excess of 50 g of fibre a day – compared to the average of 10 g of fibre which we achieve on a typical Western diet. They achieve this quantity because vegetable foods make up the major part of their diet. The UK Health Department recommends 18 g a day, and the National Cancer Institute in the USA recommends 25–35 g a day.

The significant changes that happened to the Stone Age Diet occurred in two phases. The first phase began when groups of people started to settle and build small villages. During this time they began to pen animals for a ready supply of meat. This made meat more available and it thus formed a larger proportion of the diet. At some stage the villagers started to milk their animals, to drink the milk, and eventually to make yoghurt and cheeses. For the first time man began to drink and eat dairy products regularly. No other animal on this planet has ever needed to drink milk after being weaned from its mother's breast. The great number of people who are adversely affected in different ways by the consumption of dairy products, suggests that after many millennia the human constitution has still not fully adapted to a heavy dairy diet.

Another major change which occurred was the intensive growing of grains. Up until this time, some grasses, grains or cereals would have been eaten as part of the gathering process, but the substantial reliance worldwide on intensively grown grasses has changed diets in most cultures. The obvious benefit is that it has provided a ready food supply which can feed large numbers of people. The disadvantage is that we have become heavily dependent on a few foodstuffs which dominate the diet, limit nutrient sources and often create allergies or sensitivities. These sensitivities are different from culture to culture, depending on the commonly available grain. For instance, rice is a common food sensitivity amongst the Chinese community, and corn is the greatest sensitivity creating food in the US.

The second phase happened with the gradual development in the use of chemicals as fertilisers, pesticides and herbicides, and the storage, transport and supply of foods. We now eat foods which have often taken several weeks to get from the tree or the soil onto our plates, and we eat many packaged foods which are designed to be stored for a year or more. Whilst we have not changed physically to any great degree in the last few thousand years, our diets have. The vitality of the foods we eat has changed beyond measure.

The Diet

The Stone Age Diet is favoured by many doctors and clinicians working as allergists, since it is a very pure diet which resolves many health problems. It is used as a basic elimination diet, to which foods are later introduced to see which ones the individual can or cannot tolerate. You may want to try this diet yourself if you have intractible health problems or if other elimination diets do not work for you. On the other hand, it is not the easiest of plans to follow if you want any sort of a social life.

The Stone Age Diet is very simple to implement. It involves eating foods which our ancestors are likely to have eaten, in roughly similar quantities and variety. By implication, this means that foods and drinks which are later innovations are eschewed. It is also recommended that modern-day chemicals are avoided by eating organic food and minimising exposure to household chemicals and to over-the-counter drugs (prescribed drugs should not be stopped or reduced without consulting your doctor).

The Stone Age Diet allows you to eat meat and game, fish, honey and seeds (including coconut), but these should not form more than 30 per cent of the diet. The bulk of the diet, 70 per cent in total, should consist of salad leaves, green leafy vegetables, root vegetables (potato, sweet potato, parsnips, swede, yam, carrots) and fruits (other than citrus). Buckwheat, quinoa, sago and tapioca are also allowed, as are very small quantities of oils. Bottled, non-carbonated, water is the main drink, though herbal infusions can be used. Moderate amounts of diluted fresh fruit juices are fine (though not citrus), which, along with vegetable juices, help to ring the changes.

The Stone Age Diet does not permit most grains/cereals (wheat, oats, rye, barley, corn, sweetcorn, rice, millet), dairy products (milk, cheese, yoghurt, butter), peanuts, sugar, alcohol, coffee, tea, chocolate and any other modern food innovations. All tinned, packaged, processed and convenience foods and drinks are avoided. Processed meats such as bacon, ham and patés are also excluded.

Other foods which tend to cause allergies are avoided, but can be reintroduced if, after an exclusion and reintroduction period of 14 days, it is found that they do not cause problems. These foods include chicken, eggs, nuts (though not peanuts), beetroot, soya in all forms, citrus fruit, legumes (dried or reconstituted beans, peas, pulses) and any food which you know upsets you. The best reintroduction sequence is one which tests the foods which are least likely to be a problem first, so you might try the food groups in the following sequence

1 Tap water
2 Chicken, eggs
3 Rice, millet, corn, sweetcorn
4 Citrus fruit
5 Nuts (other than peanuts)
6 Rye, barley, oats
7 Soya milk, tofu, legumes, peanuts
8 Milk (300 ml), goat's cheese, sheep's cheese, white cheese, yellow cheese, blue cheese, butter (to add to vegetables)
9 Yeast (6 brewer's yeast tablets or 2 tsp baker's yeast)
10 Wheat (wholemeal spaghetti or soda bread to avoid yeast), couscous, spelt (yeast-free), sprouted wheat (yeast-free)
11 Alcohol, sugar, beetroot, plain chocolate, tea, coffee

Introduce foods one at a time, on every alternate day. It is best to try the food in the morning, before having eaten anything else. Have a reasonable portion of the food and make a note of any reactions you have – bloating, wind, cramps, diarrhoea, headaches, nasal problems, itchiness, racing pulse, palpitations, and so on. If you are a very allergic type of person, it may be a good idea to first have just one bite of the food, wait half an hour to see if you get a reaction and then, if it is OK, eat the rest. Stay on the basic diet while you test each food. Test it on one or two days only and then, whether you have a reaction or not, avoid it until the whole testing period is finished. It is best to keep a diary of foods introduced and reactions to them during this time, as it is helpful to look back at a later date.

This is a rigorous diet which is not at all easy to follow. It may seem too strict for many people, although others may prefer the fact that they have a clear set of rules with which to work, particularly if their bloating problems are very severe. Only you will know if you are one of these people. It can also seem that this diet is quite low on starches, which can be a problem for people who get hungry easily. Having said that, given that we get too much protein on a typical Western diet, many people will find that this diet, which is based on proteins and vegetables, suits them quite well. For others, there are still starchy options such as potatoes and other root vegetables, buckwheat, quinoa, sago and tapioca, and it is as well to become familiar with preparing these. For instance, quinoa cooks in the same way as rice, and buckwheat is available as noodles and can be made into pancakes, called blinis, which freeze well.

An advantage of the Stone Age Diet is that it is also (apart from fruit consumption) a near perfect anti-candida diet, and it therefore helps to resolve bloating and other health issues which are related to an overgrowth of this yeast. It is not, however, necessary to go on such a rigorous diet just to deal with candida, and I describe an amended version later in this chapter.

One reason why the Stone Age Diet works is probably because of a component in carbohydrate foods called lectins. Lectins are proteins which bind with carbohydrates and which can cause problems by attaching themselves to particular parts of the human anatomy, such as the mucous membrane of the digestive tract, or to histamine producing mast cells which are involved in many allergies, or to blood cells, bringing about an allergic reaction. It is suggested that the gliadin in wheat gluten has a lectin-like effect which causes problems in people with coeliac disease. Lectins in foods, for instance peanuts, can also cause severe allergic reactions in some people, resulting in life-threatening anaphylactic shock (the closing up of the air passages). More subtly, lectins can cause reactions which lead to inflammation of the gut wall, and then to bloating. Dr Peter D'Adamo, author of *Eat Right 4 Your Type*, has done a lot of work on lectins and their effect on health and he claims that when people go on a lectin-free diet which corresponds with their particular physiology, toxic bowel problems resolve themselves within a short time. The measure of toxic bowel is the indican urine test. (Indican is a derivative of bacterial toxic by-products which give faeces their characteristic, not very pleasant, odour.) This ability to resolve toxic bowel problems would suggest that severe bloating problems, which are related to inflammation due to bowel bacteria imbalance, can be resolved by avoiding lectins with the Stone Age Diet, and clinically the evidence does support this.

Stone Age Diet Suggestions

Breakfasts
- Diluted apple juice. Grilled tomatoes and mushrooms
- Carrot juice. Quinoa with coconut milk
- Tropical fruit cocktail. Baked sweet potato
- Vegetable juice. Buckwheat noodles with tomatoes and onions
- Stewed fruit with ground or chopped seeds
- Banana and fruit drink. Tapioca with fruit

Light meals
- Tuna salad
- Avocado and prawns
- Jacket potato and salad
- Vegetable soup (e.g. leek, asparagus, onion, thickened with a mashed root vegetable such as swede)
- Grilled sardines with salad

• Roasted vegetables (include courgettes, red onions, aubergines, sweet peppers, garlic cloves, pumpkin, tomatoes, olives)

Main meals

• Stir-fried pork with assorted shredded vegetables (no nuts or rice)
• Cottage pie made with lean minced lamb or beef, onions, carrots and mashed parsnip with potato topping
• Fish platter with assorted grilled vegetables
• Rabbit casserole with celery, carrots, peppers and mushrooms
• Pork with apple sauce and roasted parsnips and celeriac
• Pheasant, partridge or venison with vegetables
• Main course salad
• Peppers stuffed with vegetables and diced lamb/beef/fish

Convenience options

There are very few convenience options on the Stone Age Diet, and success largely depends upon being prepared to cook meals from scratch and on being able to plan ahead by taking your own meals and snacks when necessary. Ignoring for the moment that one of the recommendations is to eat pesticide-free organic foods, there are a few easy options which you can fall back on when you need to:

• Organic, freshly pressed apple juice, and other juices.
• Cold cuts from the delicatessen counter of the supermarket. Add to this a pre-prepared salad with oil and lemon dressing.
• Cold salmon and other unsmoked fish which is not tinned

(though you may want to relax this rule eventually) eaten with pre-prepared salad or vegetables.

● Packets of sunflower seeds can be carried around as snacks.

● You may be able to buy baked potatoes from your sandwich shop – top with tuna with no mayonnaise, but use a little olive oil and lemon.

● Fruit is the best fast-food around.

● An avocado pear, eaten like a fruit, can work wonders when you need something calorie dense to carry you through. Avocados also jazz up many other dishes.

● Look out for freshly prepared vegetable and meat based soups which do not contravene your dietary restrictions.

● Some of the supermarkets and chain stores have excellent prepared salads which will fit your plan, for example carrot and sultana salad or green salads. Add these to some cold cuts or fish fillets and you have a delicious meal.

PLAN 3: STOP FOODS FIGHTING

Food combining is the general name given to programmes where meals consist of mainly starch foods or protein foods. This way of eating has some enthusiastic advocates, and it certainly does seem to work for a significant number of people. Possible benefits include a reduction, or elimination, of bloating problems such as water retention, stomach distension and wind. It is also often the case that people who normally find it difficult to lose weight can do so when they adopt the Stop Foods Fighting approach.

Many different diets claim to be 'new', and recent diets, which are all food combining of one sort or another, include *Fit For Life*, *The Montignac Diet*, *Sugar Busters!* and *The Kensington Diet*. They are all twists on an old theme. By virtue of the fact that these regimes suggest that meals be protein and vegetable based, and that foods which combine proteins and starches, which are also high in sugars, are not eaten (for example, milk and flour in biscuits or cakes), it follows that there is an automatic balancing of blood sugar levels which helps with weight loss. These diets certainly seem to suit some people and there are also some good 'straight' food combining books available, which I list in **Resources** page 198.

The basic principle centres on the fact that the digestive tract has different areas which are either acidic for protein digestion, or alkaline for starch digestion. It is suggested that mixed meals will slow up digestion as starches inevitably hang around while the proteins are being digested, and similarly any undigested proteins will slow up the subsequent digestion of starch. A significant number of people who adopt food combining as a way of eating, find that they benefit digestively. Fruits, which go through the first part of the digestive tract very quickly, if they are not in the presence of other foods, are eaten separately.

Food combining is also sometimes called the Hay Diet, after Dr William Hay who, in 1911, devised this way of eating and, along the way, cured himself of Bright's disease, high blood pressure and a dilated heart, at the same time dropping his weight from 102 kg to 77 kg in only three months. He subsequently used it with his patients for a range of other ailments. He described his diet as 'eating fundamentally', in other words eating only foods that he believed nature intended. He explained the clearing up of his symptoms as being due to a reversal of the condition which led to them, the 'condition' being an accumulation of acidic end products of metabolism in quantities greater than the body was able to tolerate. It is also interesting to note that people who need to put on weight can often do so with this regime over time, indicating that this way of eating does seem to balance body chemistry in some people.

The basic rules of the Stop Foods Fighting approach is a simplified version of the Hay or food combining system – without all the difficult rules and exceptions. Three types of meals can be eaten:

- PROTEIN with vegetables
- STARCH with vegetables
- FRUIT meals

Foods which are principally proteins should not be eaten at the same meal as foods which are principally starches. To qualify for being principally protein a food has to be more than 20 per cent protein and, similarly, principally starchy foods have to be more than 20 per cent starch. Either of these food groups can be combined with 'neutral' foods at meals. This basic rule means that a meal may consist of meat with vegetables or salad, or rice with vegetables or salad, but not meat AND rice with vegetables or salad.

Protein foods are: meat, poultry, fish, eggs, cheese, milk, soya, nuts, seeds, yoghurt

Starchy foods are: potato, bread, pasta, rice, oats, rye, barley, sweetcorn, honey and sugars

Neutral foods: can be combined with either proteins or starch based meals and include green leafy vegetables, avocados, red/yellow vegetables and root vegetables (but not potatoes), sprouted legumes, sprouted seeds, sprouted grains, butter and oils (avoid margarine), egg yolks, cream (full fat).

Other points

- The sharp-eyed will immediately notice that the principles of food combining ignore the fact that some foods naturally contain a combination of proteins and starches, for example legumes, nuts and seeds, and yet we are surely designed to digest them? According to the Hay system, however, the only naturally occurring incompatible foods, containing proportions of both proteins and starches that make them difficult to digest, are unsprouted legumes, peas, beans, lentils and peanuts, see **Beanz Meanz Wind**, page 173. When they are sprouted their nature changes to that of highly beneficial green plants that can be combined with either starches or proteins. Indeed, it is perfectly possible to make dishes such as hummus and Mexican bean dishes from sprouted beans.

- Vegetables, salads and fruits should form the bulk of the diet. Only wholefoods should be eaten, and refined foods, sugar, processed fats, such as margarines, and artificially coloured and sweetened foods and drinks, such as fruit squash, avoided completely.

- It can be tempting with starch based meals to eat more bread or pasta, but this can be a problem for those with a gluten grain intolerance. It is important, therefore, to concentrate on starches which are less likely to be troublesome, such as potatoes, rice and corn, or to eat other root vegetables, or sprouted legumes which are filling. On the other hand, it is not unusual for people with gluten grain intolerances to find that food combining allows them to tolerate gluten grains more successfully.

- There is a danger that fruits can be avoided altogether, and this is a shame because they are such a useful food, providing antioxidants, fibre and enzymes. If you decide to follow this diet, it may be best to eat a fruit based breakfast to ensure that you get your daily quota.

● Alcohol is a carbohydrate and so should only be consumed with carbohydrate based meals. Having said this, alcohol, coffee and tea are such strong stimulants that they are best kept to a bare minimum on this regime.

Planning your day

The key to successful food combining is to have a plan. Know what suits you in terms of organisation and make the rules fit your life. Here are some tips.

● You may find it easiest to have a 'neutral' breakfast (i.e. fruit juice or a fruit plate and then grilled tomatoes and mushrooms and vegetable juice), followed by a 'starch' lunch (i.e. baked potato and salad) and then finally a 'protein' evening meal (i.e. chicken and vegetables).

● Other people find that it is easier to have a 'starch' day, followed by a 'protein' day, thereby ensuring that there is no clash with snacks taken between meals.

● Before you go to a restaurant, consider ahead of time what sort of meal you are likely to have. You can predict fairly closely what a menu in an Italian, Indian, Chinese or Middle Eastern restaurant is likely to offer, so decide what you might order before you go. This helps to avoid getting sidetracked with foods which are likely to fight in your digestive tract. For example, in an Italian restaurant, have salad or vegetable soup with Parmesan, followed by fish or chicken with vegetables. In an Indian restaurant have chicken tikka with spinach and tomato curry. In a Chinese restaurant have mixed vegetables with mushrooms and seaweed with rice or noodles. In a Middle Eastern restaurant have yoghurt dip with crudités followed by lamb kebabs and vegetables. You get the idea.

● At a private party you have a few choices. You could notify your host in advance that you are aiming to eat simply – say fish and vegetables. If this is not an option, then you could accept more of the foods which fit your plan, and less of those that do not – you may feel self-conscious, but the reality is that most hosts and guests will not notice if the evening is lively enough. Desserts often present a problem but, if you have had a protein based meal and are not dairy intolerant, you can always accept a little cheese. And life is not always perfect – you always have the option to go off the rails . . . Just get back on them the next day!

Examples of food-combined meals
. . . .

● Fish, chicken or game grilled or baked with lemon, wine, garlic and herbs with two or three fresh vegetables (no starches allowed).

● Omelette with vegetable fillings, e.g. leek and mushroom, peppers and tomatoes, spinach and onions or a hard cheese and mixed herbs. Side salad. (No potatoes or bread allowed.)

● Wholewheat pasta or couscous with tomato, onion, peppers or other vegetables. (No cheese or meat allowed.) If you are wheat intolerant use pastas based on other grains, such as corn, rice or buckwheat, which are available from health food shops.

● Guacamole, salsa and mushrooms-à-la-Gréque from the deli counter of your supermarket, crudités (with whole-meal pitta bread, rye crackers or oatcakes if you are not gluten grain intolerant).

- Baked potato with coleslaw in vinaigrette, chargrilled peppers and other vegetables.
- Sandwich (rye bread, wholewheat bread, or gluten-free bread) with avocado, tomato, spring onion and olive oil and herb dressing.
- Buckwheat noodles with garlic, sun-dried tomato, capers, olives and red peppers.
- Quinoa with grilled vegetables, or vegetable tajhine.

PLAN 4: ANTI-CANDIDA PROGRAMME

To eliminate an overgrowth of candida, it is most effective to combine a dietary programme together with anti-candida supplements. Start with the diet for two or three weeks, and then continue with the diet while you add in supplements. The length of time it takes in total to resolve the problem largely depends on how bad the candida is in the first place, how meticulous you are about following the anti-candida plan, and how efficiently your immune system is working. The most important foods to avoid are sugar, refined carbohydrates, yeast and alcohol. In the same way that sugar is used to make yeast grow to expand bread dough or to ferment alcohol, too much sugar in the diet can increase the number of yeast organisms resident in the bowels, including *Candida albicans*. If you are pregnant, or planning a pregnancy, you should not attempt an anti-candida programme as there is no research available on the effect of candida 'die-off' on the developing foetus. On the other hand, if you plan to get pregnant in the future, and are sure that you will not do so while you are on an anti-candida programme, then dealing with a candida problem can only be beneficial for any future pregnancy.

Anti-Candida Diet

The whole point of an anti-candida diet is to starve the candida of the foods it thrives on.

Foods you can enjoy: meat, poultry, fish, eggs, tofu, vegetables, beans, pulses, oils, yoghurt, cottage cheese, fresh nuts, fresh seeds and wholegrains without yeast (wholemeal soda bread, wholemeal scones, oatcakes, porridge, rye crackers, brown rice, rice cakes, sugar-free muesli, etc). Usually fruits which are not excessively sweet are allowed, such as green apples and green pears. If the candida is extremely bad then even these fruit may be best avoided.

Foods to be avoided: alcohol, sugar (sucrose, maltose, lactose, dextrose, glucose), foods containing yeast (bread, cheese, soya sauce), processed meats and other processed foods, grains (if you are sensitive to them, but use in moderation otherwise), all dried fruits, most fresh fruits which are very sweet. Vinegars and mushrooms are also avoided on strict anti-candida diets, but may be tolerated by some people. Quorn is a mycoprotein, made from mushrooms, and needs to be avoided at the same time. Some people may also be sensitive to cooked carrots and parsnips as they become quite sugary, and also to the squash family (cucumber and courgettes) as they convert quickly to sugar in the gut.

It is best to go on a strict diet using only the first list of foods for two or three months and then slowly to introduce one food at a time from the second list to work out if you are sensitive to it – some people can tolerate fruits, mushrooms or dairy products in moderation, for instance, while others cannot. The major foods which should not be reintroduced until you are sure the candida is well under control are alcohol and sugar, and then only in moderation.

Medication

The fastest way to eliminate candida is by taking a preparation such as Nystatin or Diflucan. Different drugs have different applications, and some will be appropriate for one lot of people, but not for others. Medication can induce such a fast 'die-off' of the candida yeast that the level of toxic by-products can be unacceptably high, causing a range of unpleasant symptoms. Medication can also have side effects, including local burning with some pessaries, nausea, vomiting and diarrhoea, especially if used in high doses. Pharmaceutical preparations are not always effective as candida can be very resistant, and relying on them in the absence of adjusting diet often leads to disappointment. Natural anti-candida agents take longer and may need to be continued for three to six months, but they are more gentle, and encourage a slower die-off, producing less toxic by-products. Anti-candida agents, medication or natural, are not advised during pregnancy.

Natural Anti-Candida Agents

It is important, when using strong anti-fungals, particularly in supplement form, that you follow the recommended doses. If you begin to feel worse, perhaps more tired, it is possible that this is caused by toxins being released from the candida as it dies. This is referred to as die-off. Die-off does not affect everyone taking anti-fungals, but the few who experience it can find it unpleasant. If the die-off exceeds a sensible comfort zone, do not be a martyr, reduce the dose of your anti-fungals. The herb milk thistle (silymarin) and cloves can be helpful, as they decrease the die-off effect of candida. Milk thistle also supports the liver to help it deal with the extra toxic load. These are the most popular natural anti-candida agents.

Caprylic acid This is a short-chain fatty acid, extracted from coconuts, which is present in breast milk. As caprylic acid is readily absorbed by the intestines it should be taken in a time-release formula so that it reaches the lower intestines and the bowels. One 400 mg capsule is taken three times a day, between meals. Higher and lower strengths are available and can be used, depending on a person's sensitivity to the die-off.

Garlic Best taken raw on salads or crushed and mixed with olive oil as a dressing for vegetables. Supplements are available, but do not be tempted to use the odourless variety as the active compounds have been removed. Whole peeled garlic cloves can also be used as a vaginal suppository if vaginal thrush is present, but be careful not to scratch the surface of the clove, or cut across the root base, as it then stings unmercifully.

Olive oil Contains a type of monounsaturated fat, oleic acid, which limits the yeast's ability to convert into the fungal form. Extra virgin oil is always the best choice and although it is fine to cook with it at low temperatures, it is best not to overheat it as it loses some of its active ingredients. Use it on salads, or drizzle on baked potatoes or other vegetables.

Ginger, oregano, basil, rosemary and thyme Incorporating these in your meals must make this the tastiest way to help control a candida overgrowth. They are a helpful add-on, but really need to be used alongside other stronger anti-fungals. Oregano oil supplements are available and may be even more effective than the more popular caprylic acid. Take 0.6 mg in two or three divided doses daily.

Biotin A member of the B-complex, 200 mcg of yeast-free biotin, three times daily (a total of 600 mcg) can help to prevent the conversion of the yeast-like form of candida into the invasive mycelioid form. Biotin is sometimes included in garlic capsules, especially formulated for candida treatment.

Pau d'arco (La pacho or taheebo) A South American tree which contains two compounds, Lachopol and xyloidine, which have a strong anti-fungal effect. Supplements are available.

Berberine This strengthens the immune system, which is often at a low ebb in those who have candida, and is an effective anti-microbial, including anti-fungal. It is found naturally in goldenseal, Oregon grape root and barberry, all of which are available as supplements.

Grapefruit seed extract This was discovered by a doctor and Einstein Laureate physicist who, when gardening, noticed that the grapefruit seeds thrown on the compost heap did not rot. He discovered that this bitter substance had very potent anti-microbial properties. There has been tremendous success in treating candida with grapefruit seed extract, which is available in liquid and capsule form. A dose of 75–150 mg is taken three times daily (a total of 225–450 mg).

Pseudowintera colorata The active ingredient of this New Zealand shrub leaf is polygodial, which is an anti-fungal agent. Exceeding the recommended one capsule daily is unwise as it can cause a strong die-off reaction.

Propolis This extract from bee pollen exhibits anti-fungal properties and can help against candida.

Other measures
. . . .

As candida can cause a loss of nutrients because of malabsorption, it is important to take a daily multivitamin and mineral supplement which is sufficiently high-dose to top up levels again. In particular, vitamin B6 and magnesium can be severely depleted. Make sure, however, that any B-complex you buy is yeast free. Vitamin C, 3 g taken daily, can also help to support the immune system. Acidophilus helps to discourage candida and can be taken during the main anti-candida programme as well as afterwards. During an active attack of thrush or cystitis, it can also be helpful to drink sugar-free cranberry juice, or to take cranberry supplements. Douche in warm water with added apple cider vinegar and tea tree oil (1 quart water, 2 tbsp apple cider vinegar, a few drops of tea tree oil). Avoid intercourse at this time so as not to infect your partner. For suggested brands of all the supplements see **Resources**, page 193.

CHAPTER TWENTY-THREE

A – Aid Digestion

In Eliminate the Cause you have addressed by far the most difficult aspects of bringing your bloating under control. The remainder of the programme is no less important but can be thought of as simply developing the basic theme.

Here we look at giving your digestive tract a chance to do its job efficiently by examining when and how you eat, the possibility of using digestive enzymes if they are deficient, and other digestive aids.

HOW DO YOU EAT?

The immediate answer which comes to mind may be 'with my mouth, of course', but there is more to it than that. What is the *atmosphere* in which you eat? *When* do you eat? *How much* do you eat? It is worth reflecting for a few moments on how you go about this daily ritual, and assessing whether some changes would be desirable.

● First and foremost it is important to relax when eating. Nervous tension at meal times limits the digestion and means that while you may be eating healthily, you may not be getting the best out of your food, nutritionally speaking. In practical terms this may mean taking time out to prepare food in a relaxed environment, instead of grabbing something in a rush. It may mean moving away from your desk to eat your lunch in a park or in a staff room. It may mean taking the phone off the hook and laying the table nicely.

- Chewing your food well is vital. Asking your stomach and intestines to do the job that your mouth is meant to do is asking too much. Chewing stimulates gastric and pancreatic juices and breaks down the surface area of the food sufficiently to allow these juices to do their job properly.

- You may be bloating because you are eating large portions, and the distended feeling in your stomach may be the result of your digestive capacity being unable to cope with the size of the meals (and, of course, if you are eating large quantities you may also find that you are putting on fat-weight as well as bloating). You may find that you are better off eating five or six small snacky meals a day – or grazing – rather than eating three large 'square' meals a day, which may be harder to digest.

- Conversely, some people find it easier to eat twice a day. Once mid-morning and once mid-afternoon, thus also ensuring that food is not eaten too late at night and left 'sitting' in the system. There are no rules about which system is best. Most people know instinctively which is best for them, and which relaxes their digestion and reduces bloating most.

DIGESTIVE SUPPLEMENTS

If your digestion is disturbed and you are not digesting meals adequately you may want to try a course of digestive supplements. Usually it is sufficient to simply eliminate foods which have been disturbing digestion, or to follow a plan such as Stop Foods Fighting. However, if there is still some residual discomfort, or symptoms such as loose stools or constipation, a course of digestive enzymes can make a huge difference by promoting better nutrient absorption. Sufficient pancreatic enzymes are critical for ensuring that food molecules are broken down enough in order not to provoke food allergies. The large undigested molecules, called IPBs (incomplete protein breakdown products), can cause allergic reactions, and can overtax the immune system, producing inflammation and other immune reactions. Food allergies are also major contributors to bloating. Sometimes digestive enzyme supplements are needed to break the vicious downward spiral and start the upturn.

Fat digesting supplements Bile emulsifies fat, in much the same way as washing-up liquid breaks down the fat globules on greasy dishes and allows them to mix with the water. When the bile has done this job, the enzymes can get on with their task of digesting the fat, ready for absorption across the villi. The fat digesting enzymes are called lipases and low levels can be a player in poor absorption of the healthy essential fats as well as the fat soluble vitamins.

It is common for people to feel that they have fat digestion problems and that they cannot tolerate rich, creamy or fatty dishes. On closer questioning they will readily agree that they are quite happy eating oils in salad dressings or, for instance, oily fish. Since all fats are digested in the same way, this would suggest that they don't have problems digesting fat, *per se*, but that it is the combination of foods which is causing the problem.

If fat digestion problems are suspected it may be a good idea to try supplementing with a broad-spectrum digestive enzyme which contains the fat digesting enzyme lipase. The fat emulsifier, lecithin, can also be used, and is especially useful for those who have had their gall bladder removed. Lecithin is a fat itself, but it is a fat which emulsifies other fats. It is pleasant tasting and can be bought in granules which can be sprinkled on cereals, in soups, stews or in desserts.

HCl (hydrochloric acid) supplements If you think that you have low stomach acid levels then supplements of HCl are readily available. If you take them and get a burning sensation, stop them immediately, though this is extremely rare. Another way of testing whether they might be inappropriate because your stomach acid levels are already too high is to drink some slightly diluted lemon juice on an empty stomach to see if it creates an acid sensation in your stomach. Do not take HCl supplements on an empty stomach as they are too acidic on their own and need to be taken with meals – also do not be tempted to chew them! Once you have had a couple of mouthfuls of food, then you can take your HCl. Betain hydrochloride with pepsin provides a natural source of HCl. Take one or two 10 mg capsules with each meal, depending on the size of the meal, to see if it makes a difference to your digestion. If it does not improve, build up slowly to a maximum of five capsules with each meal. If you get a warm or burning sensation this indicates that you have exceeded the correct dosage for your needs, and you should immediately drink a glass of milk, or a solution comprised of one teaspoon of baking soda dissolved in water. Cut back the number of capsules at the next meal. Use them for at least three months, while making positive changes to your diet. After that time, you should be able to reduce, and stop, your use of them. This is because the programme of HCl use should have boosted mineral absorption from foods, especially zinc, which is instrumental in restoring the stomach's ability to produce its own HCl. Some people, especially those in their sixties or older, may need to continue use indefinitely.

Vinegar You can also raise stomach acidity levels by using vinegar – though this takes a degree of dedication! Put one teaspoon of vinegar in water and drink this concoction with each meal. Slowly increase the quantity of vinegar up to a maximum of ten teaspoons. If a burning sensation is experienced you can immediately neutralise the acidity level by drinking a glass of milk, or by taking a teaspoon of baking soda dissolved in water. If this happens then you must cut back on the level of vinegar at the next meal. Over time, you should be able to cut back on the vinegar levels as your overall digestion, and therefore HCl production, improves.

Helicobacter pylori If low stomach acidity has resulted in an infection of *Helicobacter* (the 'ulcer bug'), then this will need treating. First it must be diagnosed by your doctor, as treatment will entail a course of antibiotics. It is important to be retested a couple of months later, because antibiotic treatment is not always totally successful. If you do have to take antibiotics then review the information in **Establish a Healthy Environment**, page 165, for details on how to replenish healthy bowel bacteria. Research has shown that high doses of vitamin C are effective in eradicating a significant proportion of *Helicobacter* cases, and helping to restore stomach acidity. Levels of 10 g per day (taken in 3-5 divided doses) should be maintained for two to three months, eventually tailing this dose off to a maintenance level of 1–3 g daily. Powdered vitamin C is the easiest, and least expensive, way to accomplish this, and it can be added to water or fruit juices.

Digestive enzymes Digestive enzymes can be taken just before, during or just after a meal, whichever is convenient. Do not rely on them for the long term, as they can encourage the pancreas to become lazy. The point about using them is to break the downward spiral, as suggested previously, create better nutrient absorption to promote improved health, and simultaneously improve the diet to the point when you can be weaned off them. Take two to five capsules, depending on the size of the meal.

There are many different types of digestive enzyme compounds and it is usually best to go for a good broad-spectrum supplement which contains amylase, protease, lipase, lactase, cellulase. See **Resources**, page 193.

Other uses for digestive enzymes There are some other interesting methods of taking digestive enzymes for various alternative purposes. These theories have not been substantiated with medical trials, but this does not mean that they do not work. They all centre on taking digestive enzymes away from meals – in other words not taking them to digest your food. The theory is that digestive enzymes taken away from meals will then be able to 'digest' unwanted matter in the digestive tract, and further afield in the body. The theory goes on to say that any surplus enzyme activity is used by the body to manufacture other enzymes – so you are effectively replenishing your enzyme reserve.

Digestive enzymes certainly work well at stopping food poisoning in its tracks. If you feel a stomach upset is on its way following a suspect meal, take around ten enzyme capsules to digest the multiplying bacteria in the stomach. This can be a very useful trick when eating in developing countries where tummy upsets are a constant threat to visitors. I have also found it helpful to take digestive enzymes to 'digest' unhealthy mucus, for example three or four enzyme tablets between meals, in addition to those with meals, to help to dissolve mucus in the respiratory tract.

HELPFUL HERBALS

There are some herbal preparations, many of which make delicious teas, which can aid digestion. Herbs must not be taken if pregnant or breastfeeding without the advice of a qualified herbal practitioner.

Dandelion tea This is a mildly diuretic drink which can help to reduce water retention and bloating. Do not drink dandelion tea in great quantities as it can also be mildly laxative. Take five to six dandelion leaves and remove any stems. Break the leaves into pieces and place them in a mug. Steep in boiling water and leave for 5–10 minutes. Strain and discard the leaves and drink. You can sweeten it with a teaspoon of honey. You can also buy dandelion supplements. Dandelion root, available as a coffee alternative, helps to stimulate bile action.

Fennel or anise water Fennel is the classic base for gripe water, but it is not limited in its usefulness to babies – adults can benefit as well. It helps to dispel trapped wind. Crush 1 tsp of fennel seeds or aniseeds and cover with boiling water in a mug. Leave to steep for 20 minutes, strain out the seeds and drink the liquid.

Liquorice This is one of the oldest medicinal herbs and it tastes nice as well. An infusion is made by adding 25 g of bruised root, with the bark removed, to 500 ml of boiling water, which is then allowed to cool. Drink a wine glassful three times a day. It is very useful for ulcers and gastric catarrh. A strong decoction of the root can help to relieve constipation. Do not use liquorice if you suffer from raised blood pressure as it can increase fluid retention.

Mint and peppermint These two have been used for centuries, at least as far back as the Romans, to help combat nausea, flatulence and vomiting, and have also been used as an infant's cordial. Peppermint oil capsules have, in addition, been used to relieve IBS, and have proved helpful against candida. Tea bags are readily available, or you can grow mint easily on a windowsill.

Ginger A few slices of ginger, or 1/2 a teaspoon of dried ginger, steeped in boiling water and left until it is cool

enough to drink will help to dispel trapped wind. Ginger
tea can also be very soothing for heartburn, and can help
to relieve griping pains.

Aloe vera Used for over 2000 years for the relief of
inflammation and for healing. It contains mucopoly-
saccharides which have been shown to be highly beneficial
to the integrity of the digestive tract. It is also used to heal
stomach and duodenal ulcers. It is not advised during
pregnancy.

Milk thistle The active component of this herb is silymarin,
which has been shown to inhibit liver damage, while at the
same time enhancing protein manufacture by the liver.
It also has liver specific antioxidants and increases the
production by the liver of the important antioxidant
enzymes superoxide dismutase (SOD) and glutathione
peroxidase. These enzymes help protect against toxins
which may damage the liver, and also better enable the
liver to deal with toxins which need to be neutralised.
Supporting the liver can also help to balance hormone
levels. Take six 100 mg capsules of standardised extract
daily – two with each meal.

Slippery elm This favourite of the herbal cabinet is soothing
to the mucous membranes of the digestive tract – the
name describes it well. It is useful for any inflammation or
ulceration of the digestive tract, particularly as it is
non-toxic. You can buy capsules, or you can make tea by
simmering a teaspoon of slippery elm bark in two cups of
water for 20 minutes and then straining. You may want to
sweeten this tea with honey. Drink freely.

Meadowsweet I love the name of this herb, which is also
known as queen of the meadow. In the past it was used in
beer-making, and you can often find it in fields near inns
where it has self-seeded. Meadowsweet soothes inflamed

mucous membranes, slows the motility of the digestive tract when diarrhoea is present and, because of its mild astringency, is useful for indigestion. It also helps to normalise acid secretions in the stomach. Make a tea by steeping one or two teaspoons of the herb in a cup of boiling water for 10 minutes. Sweeten with honey if desired. Drink three cups daily. You can also combine it with liquorice and dandelion roots for an all-round digestive tonic.

Marshmallow This is another soothing herb, which is used to calm an irritated or inflamed digestive tract, particularly in cases of colitis and gastritis. In the past, it was frequently grown in gardens because of its curative properties. To make an infusion, add 25 g of leaves to 500 ml of boiling water and allow to cool. Strain and add a little honey or orange juice. Take 50 ml three or four times a day. The dried root, which can be bought in health food shops, produces a mucus-like substance when boiled which can help to replace healthy mucus lining the digestive tract. It can be added to slippery elm, which complements it.

Rose tea Both the petals and the leaves are rich in tannins which can help to protect the lining of the gut from irritation and infection. The tannins can also help to stem both diarrhoea and constipation, and have a mild cleansing action on the liver. Rose petal tea is superb if you have a stomach or bowel infection, and can help to re-establish friendly bowel bacteria. Make the tea by steeping petals and/or leaves in boiling water for 10 minutes. Make sure you do not use ingredients from trees which have been sprayed. Avoid using in pregnancy, until the last two weeks, as it has a stimulating effect on the uterus.

QUICK FIXES FOR WATER RETENTION

There are a number of remedies, herbal and nutrient, which can help alleviate a bloating crisis caused by water retention, particulary one linked to hormone imbalance. There really is no substitute for addressing other dietary issues, such as food sensitivities and excess stimulants, but if you need a quick fix, give some of the following a go.

● Remember to always drink sufficient water, as fresh water clears out stagnant water. Six to eight large glasses daily can make all the difference.

● Natural diuretics are gentle and do not have the negative side effects of medicinal diuretics which can disturb the fine balance of the detoxification systems, and which do not get to the root of the problem anyway. One of the best to try is ten cups of camomile tea in a day to shift water retention.

● Dandelion tea is also effective and you can use young leaves from unsprayed dandelions in your weed patch. Wear gloves when you pick them! If gardening is not your forte you can take dandelion supplements, see **Resources**, page 193.

● Two capsules of celery seed extract, and 1 g of vitamin C (as potassium ascorbate) three times daily helps to encourage lymph drainage.

● For lower leg swelling use gotu kola. This herb stimulates circulation in the lower limbs and increases lymph drainage.

● For puffy ankles, herbal creams are available which contain anti-inflammatory herbs such as butcher's broom and elderflower, as well as soothing compounds such as witch hazel and horse chestnut. See **Resources**, page 193.

- Magnesium 400–600 mg daily can really help PMS-related bloating.
- Vitamin B6 is a natural diuretic and 50 mg daily along with a B-complex can help.
- Concentrated globe artichoke supplements aid liver function and can help if bloating is likely after an indulgent night out!

CHAPTER TWENTY-FOUR

S – Solve the Damage

A digestive system which has been under continued assault from foods which do not agree with it, toxic by-products of bacterial overgrowth, or possibly candida, will probably have sustained some damage to its basic fabric. Much can be done to encourage healing of the digestive tract and, if this is done successfully, there is less chance that the problems will recur at a later date.

During the time that you are working on healing the gut wall it is necessary to continue to avoid foods which you have identified as being triggers for reactions you have experienced in the past. If you find it very difficult to avoid these foods totally, you may be able to tolerate them on a rotation basis, as outlined previously. Remember that the more you eat foods which are disruptive, the longer the healing of the lining of your gut wall is likely to take, and the more protracted the whole treatment phase is going to be. In addition to avoiding foods which you know to be your particular downfall, remember that it is also necessary to restrict alcohol, and over-the-counter pain and anti-inflammatory medication. These have a particularly detrimental and direct effect on the gut wall. You would also be well advised to focus on stress management techniques if you feel that continuous stress could be a factor in your health problems. Some useful books are listed in **Resources**, page 198.

Repairing the damage to the digestive tract means healing any possible excess gut permeability, re-establishing healthy villi lining the gut wall, and eliminating inflammation along the length of the digestive tract.

SUPPLEMENTAL BENEFITS

Some supplements have been shown to speed up the healing of the gut wall considerably. If you are opposed to taking supplements, vitamins, minerals, herbs and other nutrients, you should still, over time, be able to heal the gut wall, but a bit of judicious help can prove very useful indeed. Inflammation of the gut wall frequently means that carrier proteins, which transport nutrients across the gut wall, are unable to be secreted and this severely compromises absorption. By reducing inflammation, correct absorption of nutrients from food may be restored, reducing the need for supplements.

It is always a good idea to base any supplement programme on a good quality multi-vitamin and mineral. All nutrients work together and by so doing you will provide a broad spectrum of essential vitamins and minerals which can help specific therapeutic doses of particular nutrients to work most effectively. Once you have done this, the supplements listed below can help to heal the gut wall. There are some specific, and well designed, products which combine some of these nutrients in their formulations, making it easier to take a number of them in one go. See **Resources**, page 193 and **Appendix II**.

Vitamin A Necessary for the healing of mucous membranes, vitamin A is available in the diet from liver, cod-liver oil, egg yolks, full fat dairy produce, herrings and mackerel. Vitamin A can also be made in the body from beta-carotene, which is found in leafy green vegetables and orange-coloured fruits and vegetables. It is helpful to supplement between 7,500 ius and 15,000 ius (international units) while aiming to heal the lining of the digestive tract. Diabetics and those with low thyroid function in particular have trouble converting beta-carotene into vitamin A and can benefit from supplementation. Vitamin A is not advised in excess of 6,000 ius if pregnant and taking more than this level should be avoided if you are planning a pregnancy.

Vitamin C This inexpensive and much researched nutrient is used to build collagen and is therefore very important for repairing mucous membranes. It is also an antioxidant and potent detoxifier, helping to flush toxins out of the body. Food sources are all fruits, and most vegetables, especially citrus fruits, kiwis, strawberries and cabbage. Supplementing a non-acidic form, such as magnesium ascorbate, calcium ascorbate or Ester-C, means that it is unlikely to disturb the digestive tract, and a total of 2,000–5,000 mg (2-5 gms) daily is recommended in divided doses throughout the day. Some people may experience a loosening of the bowels, though this is rare, and is not dangerous. If this happens, just cut back the dose to a level that does not produce this effect. Vitamin C is considered safe to supplement, but should be avoided by people with diagnosed haemachromatosis, and may be best avoided at levels over 1 gm if using the contraceptive pill.

Zinc Vital for all tissue building and repair, as well as for the production of enzymes and HCl, zinc is commonly deficient in the population because it is generally low in our soil and plant food. Foods rich in zinc are meat, liver, oysters, seeds, nuts, eggs, brewer's yeast, tuna and brown rice. Supplementing between 20– 30 mg during treatment for impaired gut function is highly recommended. Zinc supplementation at this level is generally very safe, but in some rare cases an isolated zinc supplement can make people feel nauseous, in which case try taking the supplement with food, or changing products.

Essential fats Ensuring that you get food sources of essential fats is, as the name implies, essential for good health. They are instrumental in healing the gut wall, and can be obtained from oily fish, fresh nuts and fresh seeds, and cold pressed, unheated, oils, including flax, walnut, sesame, sunflower and safflower. In addition to this, supplementing daily with evening primrose oil to provide 200 mg of GLA or 1 g of fish oils to provide 200 mg DHA and 150 mg EPA can be of great benefit (GLA, EPA and DHA are abbreviations for the fats these products contain and quantities should be described on the bottles).

L-glutamine This is the most abundant amino acid, or protein building block, in the body. It is used directly by the digestive tract for repairing tissue. Despite being abundant, it is considered by some experts to be 'conditionally essential', one of those conditions being disturbed digestive function. L-glutamine has been quite extensively researched and has been shown to be highly beneficial for healing damaged mucous membranes, and for conditions such as stomach ulcers, IBS and ulcerative colitis. It is available in capsule and powder form but, as fairly high doses are needed to achieve the desired effect, the powder is both more convenient and more cost effective, and it is tasteless when added to a little juice. The suggested dosage range of 5–15 g L-glutamine is generally very safe to take, but should not be taken in pregnancy, as this has not been tested. It should also not be taken by those with known kidney or liver damage.

Butyric acid This short chain fatty acid (SCFA) is normally produced by healthy bacteria in the intestines, and is used as an energy source by the surrounding cells lining the gut wall. It has been estimated that our near cousins, the great apes, derive up to 30 per cent of their dietary calories from these types of SCFAs produced in the bowel. It is fairly obvious that people with low levels of the 'good' bacteria are likely to be producing low levels of butyric acid. Butyric acid is included in some powdered formulations which are designed for healing gut walls, and also comes in capsule form. It may be easier to take the capsule form, as it has a particularly strong, and for some unpleasant, smell which can make taking the powdered form difficult. Butyric acid is generally considered safe. Take three 750 mg capsules daily, or the recommended dosage of the powdered form.

N-Acetyl glucosamine NAG is needed for the formation of proteoglycans, which glue together the gastrointestinal cells, along with collagen. Supplementing NAG can speed up the replacement of damaged gut tissues. Take two 500 mg capsules daily.

Gamma-oryzanol This is an oil found in brown rice, and increasing brown rice, or rice bran, in the diet is generally beneficial, unless you have particular problems with rice. The extracted oil is found in supplements and has been extensively researched in Japan, being one of the most frequently taken supplements there. A dose of 100 mg three times daily can be very useful for repairing the mucous membrane of the digestive tract. It is generally considered safe to supplement.

Other supplements

The following supplements are not critical for healing a damaged digestive tract, but they can be very helpful for a variety of related reasons.

Quercitin This is a potent antioxidant plant flavanoid, rich
    sources of which are onions, apples, citrus fruit and
    berries. A daily dose of 500–1000 mg can help to resolve
    many inflammatory problems.

Curcumin This is a strong anti-inflammatory compound which is found in turmeric. It has antioxidant properties and is sometime combined with boswellic acid – the two together have synergistic qualities which makes for an even more potent effect. Take two or three capsules daily.

Lecithin This is useful for emulsifying fats and is particularly needed by those with low digestive capability, liver insufficiency and gall bladder problems. It can help to ensure that essential fats are absorbed adequately from the diet. It comes in capsule and granular form. The granular form is less expensive, can be sprinkled on food, and is pleasant tasting. When liquidized into drinks with some cold-pressed oil for essential fats, it blends in completely as it emulsifies the fats into the juice or smoothie. Take two to four heaped teaspoons daily.

Vitamin B12 This vitamin is often deficient in people with low hydrochloric acid output because HCl, along with intrinsic factor, is needed for B12 absorption. Meat is the best source of B12, but cooking destroys 85 per cent of it. The only other food to contain B12 is spirulina, so vegetarians have to be sure to get it from supplements or from bacteria. The most reliable source of B12 is a healthy amount of good bacteria in the bowels. Supplementing B12 may be helpful for some people – 100–200 mcg daily using sublingual (under the tongue) liquid drops, and up to 1000 mcg can be used in cases of severe B12 depletion.

NATURAL PAIN RELIEF

One of the key recommendations for healing the gut wall is to avoid over-the-counter pain and anti-inflammatory medication. For most people this presents no problem when following a dietary exclusion programme, because they find that by avoiding the foods which triggered the symptoms they have no need of the medication. Avoid, say, the wheat and the headaches or joint pains disappear.

For some people the time taken for pain relief to come from the diet can be longer, especially in the case of arthritis or premenstrual discomfort, and the temptation to take over-the-counter (OTC) medication can be overwhelming. If you can avoid it, however, the gut wall is likely to heal that much faster. To help you, here are some possible suggestions for natural pain relief.

Cherries Twenty cherries have as many pain relief compounds as one aspirin, and can help some people.

Vitamin C This can help to reduce dependency on OTC medication quite considerably. Buying a vitamin C with added flavanoids is best (see below). Take 2,000–5,000 mgs (2–5 g) daily.

Ginger, turmeric, cayenne pepper, bioflavanoids and flavanoids These all block a chemical pathway which would normally result in inflammation. Bioflavanoids and flavanoids are found in fresh fruit and vegetables, and the best sources are green tea and dark blue/purple/red berries. Half a cup of blueberries, for instance – fresh, canned in natural juices or frozen – with your breakfast can significantly reduce inflammation.

Elderberry Decreases nerve inflammation and the pain associated with it.

Bromelain This enzyme, found in pineapples, decreases the formation of a pain inducing chemical known as kinin. It also accelerates the healing of wounds and injuries.

Ginko biloba, silymarin and boswellic acid These herbs are available in supplement form and they block an inflammatory chemical pathway. Boswellic acid, which is actually frankincense, is available as a cream, for inflammatory joint conditions, pulled muscles and tendons. It gets very hot when rubbed into the skin, so beware! Only a small amount is necessary.

L-glutamine This amino acid, described earlier, also has natural pain relief qualities, probably due to its ability to reduce the production of cytokines. Cytokines are chemicals released from white blood cells which lead to pain and inflammation.

DL-phenylalanine (DPA/DLPA) This is believed to cause the release of endorphins, the brain's own painkillers. Their effect is usually short lived but powerful. Caffeine is meant to decrease the effect of endorphins and so may make pain worse. Take 250 mg of DLPA three times daily (a total of 750 mg). If there is no benefit from this dose, it may be necessary to increase it slightly but, before doing so, take into account the fact that it does not work on everyone and there can be side effects to higher doses, including increased blood pressure, headaches and anxiety. Neither DPA nor DLPA should be used if you have high blood pressure or are pregnant.

SOOTHING SMOOTHIES

A useful way of getting concentrated sources of nutrients into the diet is to make smoothies. All you need is a blender and a juicer (the type which works on hard vegetables such as carrots). With these two pieces of equipment you can make endless delicious juices and smoothies which concentrate gut healing nutrients.

Another useful thing about making smoothies is that the supplements listed above which come in powdered form can be painlessly hidden in the mixture. You can add L-glutamine powder, vitamin C powder, cold-pressed oils and lecithin, and other liquid and powdered supplements.

The most useful fruits and vegetables to help heal the lining of the gut wall are as follows.

Carrot High in beta-carotene, which is converted into vitamin A and used to heal mucous membranes. Carrots make one of the best bases for juices to which many other vegetables and fruits can be added.

Cabbage Juiced cabbage leaves may not sound particularly palatable, but they add a delicious 'green' taste to other juices. Cabbage juice has a high glutamine content, which may account for its therapeutic gut healing effect. Around ½ cup twice daily is recommended.

Pineapple and papaya These two tropical fruits make delicious nectar-like juices that are well worth making when they are in season. If you don't want to juice them, adding them to your meals is just as beneficial. They are both potent sources of digestive enzymes, bromelain and papain, which can help to clean up debris in the digestive tract and enhance digestion. Papaya also helps to restore beneficial bacteria balance in the bowels.

Berries Any red/purple/blue berries can be added to smoothies and all of them make colourful as well as delicious drinks. The natural colouring in berries such as raspberries, blueberries, loganberries, strawberries and cherries contains substances called anthocyanidins and proanthocyanidins, which are powerful inflammation modulators. They thus help to calm inflamed digestive tissue.

Spices These can be added to smoothies to give a interesting twist. Spices such as cinnamon, ginger and turmeric provide potent anti-inflammatory compounds, as well as tasting fabulous. Be adventurous and experiment – try apple and ginger, banana and cinnamon or peach with a little turmeric.

PURGING PARASITES

If all else fails with eliminating bloating – think parasites. If by now you have not had significant relief from your bloating and have been following **Healing with E.A.S.E.** for at least eight weeks to allow for hormonal shifts, then it is possible that you may have parasites. It is wise to have them checked for before embarking on a programme to eradicate them, but not absolutely necessary. Remember that they are not always easy to detect with tests and that throughout history people have conducted regular purges of parasites. You will find it difficult to heal your gut wall once-and-for-all if there are parasites present.

The fastest way to get rid of parasites is with prescription medication from your doctor. The most commonly prescribed medication is Flagyl. However, while this option takes only a week or so to eliminate them, anti-parasite drugs can place an additional stress on the liver and the heart, and disrupt the balance in the intestines, leading to further bloating problems. Common side effects of these drugs are headaches, vomiting, diarrhoea and dizziness. If liver, heart or kidney health are a weakness for you, it may be best to seek a more natural, albeit slower, route to eliminating parasites. In any event, it is wise to use a bacterial replenishing supplement, as described in **Establish a Healthy Environment** on page 165, and to consider some additional supplements for liver and digestive tract support, if you do decide to take this route.

Anti-parasitic plant preparations have been used for many centuries and are generally safer than their chemical counterparts. People can, however, have individual reactions to herbs and some can suffer side effects. In view of this, it may be best to consult a herbalist about anti-parasitic herbs. Natural anti-parasite options are available from several nutritional and herbal supplement companies, and these supplements will contain some, or all, of the ingredients in the following list. You will need to take them for between two to six months.

It is important to recognise that eliminating parasites, whether you use medication or herbal preparations, is akin to a detoxification process, and can be accompanied by detoxification symptoms such as nausea, gastrointestinal disturbances, frequent trips to the bathroom, fever or chills, headaches, or even depression.

After the first two weeks, you may be able to use anti-parasite preparations on alternate days, or every three days, to give the parasite eggs the time to hatch. The anti-parasite agents can then be effective against the newly hatched parasites, while not overburdening your system. Do not take any anti-parasite medicine or herbs if pregnant or breastfeeding.

Herbal anti-parasite preparations

Wormwood (artemesia) As the name implies, this is an anti-parasite preparation of old. It is effective against pinworms, roundworms, and beneficial in cases of malaria. The active ingredients, the sesquiterpenes, are believed to weaken parasites' resistance, thus giving our natural defence systems the opportunity to work against them. In addition to taking supplements, you can also make a tea using 1/4–1/2 tsp of powdered leaves steeped in hot water. This can be taken twice daily, but use for short periods only. While the tea and capsules are considered safe, wormwood oil is toxic and should not be used.

Goldenseal This is an effective support for the mucous

membranes of the digestive tract and has an astringent and healing effect. The active ingredient is berberine sulphate, and goldenseal is effective against amoebas, giardia and also candida.

Pumpkin seeds These are useful against tapeworms and roundworms. Large amounts need to be eaten for them to have any real impact, up to 735 g a day for adults. They can be ground up in a clean coffee grinder and mixed with juice or sprinkled on foods. Three hours after taking them, take a tablespoon of castor oil to encourage clearance of the bowels.

Black or green walnut Useful for parasites as well as fungal infections, black walnut has been used traditionally for ringworm and athlete's foot.

Garlic This familiar herb has a remarkable range of properties – antiviral, antibacterial, anti-fungal and anti-parasitic. The active compound, alliin, is effective against entomoeba, giardia and pinworms.

Berberis Also known as barberry, berberis is a bitter, digestive stimulant, bile stimulant and liver tonic, and is used for worms together with other herbs.

Grapefruit seed extract As described in the section on candida, see page 139, grapefruit seed extract is also effective against parasitic infestations.

Colloidal silver This is an expensive product, but effective against bacterial parasites. It is important to buy a good quality colloidal silver preparation.

Other anti-parasite measures

A useful follow-up to taking anti-parasitic preparations is to use proteolytic enzymes. These enzymes are digestive enzymes which deal with proteins and, if taken between meals, instead of with them, they can digest the outer protein cuticle of parasite larvae or eggs which may be resident in the intestines. Enzyme preparations which contain papain and bromelain are effective. Fresh pineapple and papaya contain high amounts of bromelain and papain and have been eaten by the natives of Mexico for centuries to treat worm infestations.

The lining of the gut wall, the mucous membrane, is more susceptible to invasion by parasites if it is damaged. The most important vitamin for this is vitamin A. Deficiency of vitamin A is associated with impaired immune function and an inability to maintain the integrity of the mucosal surfaces of the gut lining, which leaves it wide open to colonisation. (Avoid vitamin A in pregnancy.)

Sugar in all its forms, including honey, undiluted fruit juices and jams, supplies parasites with an instantly available food, and so is best avoided if aiming to eradicate parasites. It is also possible that FOS will act as food for parasites and it should therefore be avoided if you know that you definitely have parasites.

There are some foods which have anti-parasitic properties and which can be helpful to include at every opportunity: onion, garlic, pumpkin seeds, raw cabbage, fresh pineapple and papaya and the herbs thyme, sage, cloves and turmeric.

CHAPTER TWENTY-FIVE

E – Establish a Friendly Environment

The final step is to create the right environment for continued digestive and hormonal health, and this means making sure that the bacterial occupants promote health and prevent the symptom of bloating from returning to trouble you.

SUPPLEMENTING BACTERIA

The most significant beneficial bowel bacteria are the *Bifidobacteria*, *Lactobacillus acidophilus* and *Lactobacillus bulgaricus* and the best products include all three of them. See **Resources**, page 193, for some suggested brands. Make sure that the bacteria you buy – which can come in either capsule or powdered form – have at least one billion viable organisms per dose, are within the sell-by date and have been kept refrigerated. You should then keep them in the fridge at home. Taking beneficial bacteria for two to four months at the end of your E.A.S.E. programme will significantly improve the chances of remission. You may occasionally see it written that taking beneficial bacteria supplements is a waste of time because the bacteria cannot survive the acid environment of the stomach. This is not accurate. Stomach acidity discourages the lactobacilli and bifidobacteria, but does not kill them off totally. They can survive acidity even at a pH of 1.0–1.5. There have been studies confirming this, including one in which two groups of people drank a rosehip drink, one with *Lactobacillus* and one without. There was a significant decrease in flatulence, and a better stool consistency, in the group which consumed the lactobacilli.

After a course of antibiotics most bacteria will have been wiped out of the digestive tract, irrespective of whether they are 'good' or 'bad'. Half the antibiotics produced are given to animals, and so a diet high in animal meat and dairy products will have also exposed you to a high level of antibiotics without realising it. It can take eight days for the bacteria to re-establish themselves if left to their own devices, and the bad, pathogenic bacteria tend to be more opportunistic and grow back a little faster than the good bacteria. Supplementing with bacteria immediately after finishing a course of antibiotics can help to re-establish a friendly colony of bacteria more speedily, perhaps in as little as two days. There are intensive recolonisation products available specifically designed for use after a course of antibiotics, see **Resources**, page 193. They can be followed by a more low-key, long-term addition of beneficial bacteria.

FAB FIBRE

A diet high in fibre is conducive to encouraging the correct conditions in the bowels for the growth of beneficial bacteria. The exception to this is if the fibre is of a type that causes a sensitivity reaction, as does wheat fibre in a number of people, and oat fibre in a few. Maintaining fibre levels in the diet is vital for promoting a healthy colony of bowel bacteria, and is also essential for getting rid of excess oestrogens, which contribute to water retention. This makes fibre essential in the battle against hormone induced bloating.

For optimal functioning of the digestive tract we need around 30 g of fibre a day. And yet the average intake on a typical Western diet is around 10 g a day. Dietary fibre sources are mainly fruit, vegetables, legumes, grains, nuts and seeds. Unfortunately, for most people with bloating, grains will contribute the major amount of fibre to the diet, which can be self-defeating as the grains often cause the worst digestive problems. Non-gluten grains, such as buckwheat and millet, are still excellent fibre sources. Doing a quick check of a typical day's menu can be helpful in establishing where you need to make changes. And if you need to avoid grains you can increase other sources of fibre in your diet, or slowly add supplemental fibre in a gentle, non-irritating form. One important thing to remember is that if you increase your fibre intake, you also need to increase your water, or liquid, intake. This will greatly reduce the chance of constipation resulting from a sudden increase in fibre levels.

Sources of fibre

Listed below are common sources of fibre from fresh foods. To find the fibre content of packaged foods, look on the nutrition panel which will give the amount per 100-g or 100-ml per serving. Check to see how much your serving portion actually is.

Foods which have no, or trace amounts of, fibre

meat, poultry, fish, eggs, dairy products, fats and oils, confectionery, most beverages, though vegetable or fruit juices, and soya, rice or oat milks, may contain small amounts

Foods which give around 0.5 g of fibre

100 g   tofu
50 g   asparagus, melon, pineapple, tomato

25 g   French beans, cabbage, carrots, cauliflower, celery, cherries, fresh figs, lettuce, strawberries

Foods which give around 1.0 g of fibre

2   average apricots
1   medium peach, medium plum
100 g   cooked white rice
50 g   cooked barley, rhubarb
25 g   white bread, broccoli, Brussels sprouts
15 g   blackberries, currants, chestnuts, raisins, sunflower seeds,walnuts

Foods which give around 1.5 g of fibre

100 g   cooked brown rice
50 g   swede
25 g   raw beetroot, uncooked oatmeal, peas, cooked spinach
15 g   blackcurrants, dried dates, peanuts
10 g   almonds

Foods which give around 2.0 g of fibre

1 tbsp linseeds
1/2   medium avocado pear
1   medium apple, medium banana, medium orange, medium pear
100 g   white cooked spaghetti, whole potatoes
50 g   cooked lentils, parsnips, yam
25 g   wholemeal bread, plantain, raspberries
15 g   fresh coconut

Foods which give around 3.0 g of fibre

100 g   white flour
50 g   cooked butter beans, cooked haricot beans,

cooked buckwheat (kasha), cooked chickpeas
15 g   dried figs, dried prunes

Foods which give around 5.0 g of fibre

1   medium corn on the cob
100 g   rye flour

Foods which give around 10.0 g of fibre

100 g   wholemeal flour
100 g   soya flour
100 g   cooked wholemeal spaghetti

You may notice some, seeming, anomalies in the above list. The most obvious is that white pasta has more fibre than, for instance, brown rice. Does that make it a better option? Unfortunately not. Aside from the question of sensitivity to wheat, the fibre in brown rice is much more sympathetic to the digestive system. But the main point is, that if the whole grain is used, as in brown rice or for that matter wholemeal pasta, then you also get all the associated minerals and B-vitamins. In moderation white pasta is fine, but if you eat it four times a week, then you will be missing out on the nutrients that whole grains provide.

Supplementing fibre is an easy, quick and painless way to improve the situation, and can easily be added to breakfast dishes, soups or salads. Building up slowly to two tablespoons of ground linseeds, or two teaspoons of psyllium husks, or two tablespoons of rice bran, or eight soaked prunes daily can have a marked impact in altering the colonies of the bowels for the better. When introducing fibre into your regime remember also to increase the amount of water you are drinking, if you have not already done so, to at least 2 litres daily. It is best to drink a large glass of water at the time that you are taking the added fibre, especially in the case of linseeds or psyllium.

Wheat bran This is the type of bran which is most commonly added to packaged products that claim they are high in fibre. It is also frequently bought by people to sprinkle on to their food in an attempt to increase their dietary fibre. I have always been amused by this feature of the modern Western diet – first the manufacturers sell us white bread, which constipates us, and then they sell us the bran which they extracted to add back into our foods. Marketing genius!

It should be fairly obvious that wheat bran is going to cause the same set of problems as other wheat products – sometimes more so – in people who are sensitive to wheat. These people should avoid wheat bran. Even people who do not have a wheat sensitivity are better off not relying on wheat bran as their main source of fibre. If, for any reason, you have an irritated gut wall, then wheat bran can be too aggressive and disruptive. Wheat bran is also high in phytates, which have the capacity to bind with calcium, magnesium, zinc and iron in foods and can reduce their absorption significantly.

Oat and Rice bran These are preferred sources of added bran, which you can substitute for added wheat bran. Some people react to oats by bloating, but most can happily use rice bran. Rice bran also has the advantage of containing gamma-oryzanol, a rice oil, which is highly therapeutic for the functioning of the digestive system and helps to heal the gut wall.

Linseeds Linseeds, also called flax seeds, are a wonderful source of fibre which gently expand and bulk out the stools. Linseeds are best bought whole and then ground up in a clean coffee grinder – this only takes about three seconds. You can then add them to yoghurt, soups, cereals, fruit salads, stews and baked products. You can also buy them pre-cracked, but if you do so they will contain less of the valuable omega-3 and omega-6 oils which are beneficial for maintaining a healthy gut wall. Building up slowly to two tablespoons a day of ground linseeds can work wonders for most people's digestive systems and symptoms of bloating. Make sure that you drink a large glass of water when you eat the linseeds. The people most likely to find that linseeds are troublesome are those with diverticular disease, who can find that unground linseeds may lodge in the fistulas or diverticuli.

Psyllium husks These are the ground husks of plantain. They are available either in powdered or in capsule form. They have remarkable properties and swell enormously with water or other liquids to form a thick, jelly-like, fibrous matter. They are unsurpassed at absorbing sticky mucus and loosening impacted faecal material in the bowels. In doing so, they promote very healthy bowel movements. Psyllium husks can also significantly reduce the diarrhoea to which highly lactose-intolerant people are prone. Two or three teaspoons daily of the powder, added to juices, or mixed in with yoghurt or porridge is highly effective. Though psyllium husks cause less of a 'rebound reaction' than other types of fibre, build up to this amount slowly over at least a couple of weeks if your bowels are not used to this amount of fibre.

Fruit fibre In our parents' day it was usual to be given prunes if you couldn't 'go'. Fruits such as prunes, figs, apricots, pears and raspberries are unusually high in fibre and can make the difference between being constipated and having regular, healthy bowel movements. An old wives' tale to deal with constipation is to eat four or five pears a day, which can indeed resolve the problem since this amounts to about 8–10 g of fibre daily – enough to make a significant difference in total daily fibre intake. People with candida should probably avoid dried fruit, however, and stick to the non-fruit sources of fibre during their initial treatment period.

FOS (fructo-oligo-saccharides) This is one of those rare nutritional times when you can have your cake and eat it. Or in this case, have your sugar and eat it. You can sprinkle sugar-like FOS on cereals or desserts and it will do you good instead of harm. FOS is a naturally occurring indigestible fibre which is found in many vegetables and fruits, including onions, garlic, chicory root, leeks, Jerusalem artichokes, bananas, barley, tomatoes, rye and asparagus. It has the unique ability to feed the beneficial lactobacilli and *Bifidobacteria* colonies, but not damaging organisms such as E.coli, salmonella and clostridia. The beneficial bacteria are able to do what the human body, and bad bacteria cannot: use FOS for growth and proliferation. As the damaging bacteria are suppressed by increasing colonies of *Bifidobacteria*, the levels of their toxic by-products are reduced. This in turn reduces the load placed on the detoxification activities of the liver, which frees it up to be more efficient in maintaining general health.

While there is enough FOS in foods to maintain a healthy bowel (the average good quality diet provides 2–3 g daily) there is not enough to achieve a therapeutic effect in balancing the bowel bacteria, if they are already severely out of kilter. This needs closer to 10 g daily. FOS helps to regulate the amount of time that food takes to go through the digestive tract, and increases the volume and water content of intestinal material. It has also been linked to preventing *Helicobacter pylori*, the 'ulcer' bacteria, from establishing in the stomach and upper portion of the small intestines. Additionally, FOS, along with most other dietary fibres, has the effect of balancing blood sugar levels sufficiently to be of use to diabetics as well as non-diabetics, and can have a positive effect on blood cholesterol levels as well as blood pressure. Finally, it is also being shown that FOS improves the uptake of calcium from foods.

FOS is available as an inexpensive powdered supplement which can easily be added to drinks, cereals and desserts. It tastes half as sweet as sugar but, as it is not digested or absorbed by the body, it does not add directly to calorie intake (a small number of calories are created indirectly by the action of the beneficial bacteria creating beneficial gut-feeding fats). One or two tablespoons a day is pleasant to take and highly beneficial for many people, however it is wise to start low at a teaspoon daily, and build up slowly over time. Particular care must be taken if severe bloating is already being experienced because, as with any fibre, if it is added to the diet too quickly it will make symptoms worse, and in some people it can induce further bloating. In this instance start at an even lower level of 1/4 teaspoon and build up very slowly.

It is, however, a good idea to have a short, two-week course of bacteria supplements before starting FOS in order to ensure that there are some *Bifidobacteria* there for the FOS to encourage. When choosing a FOS make sure that it is 95 per cent FOS and is manufactured by a reputable company. FOS is engineered either from sucrose or from vegetable sources such as Jerusalem artichokes. Both sources are equally good.

BEANZ MEANZ WIND

Beans are an excellent source of both soluble and insoluble fibre, as well as sitosterols, which help to stabilise blood cholesterol levels. Beans and other legumes provide just the right environment for healthy bowel bacteria to proliferate. And it is healthy bowel bacteria which help to finally break down the carbohydrates in legumes, which means that they have a less 'explosive' effect. So here we have a classic chicken and egg situation: if you eat beans and tend to get windy, then it probably means that you have an imbalance of bowel bacteria, and the best way to remedy this is to eat more beans! Realistically, though, this is likely to cause wind and discomfort for people with bad digestive problems, and these people should therefore stick to sprouted beans and pulses (see the end of this section). However, by the time you have followed all the advice in this book, your digestion should be well on the way to being healthy and slowly introducing beans into your regime can only be a good thing.

Beans contain carbohydrates called raffinose and stachyose which are often not split efficiently. They also contain other compounds, such as phytic acid and protease inhibitors, which are difficult to digest. Soaking beans for a significant amount of time before cooking them can go a long way towards reducing the gassy effect – indeed you can see the gas bubbles rising to the top of the water. It is best to change the water several times over a 12–24 hour period before cooking them. If you then freeze the home-cooked beans this will further help to decrease the flatu-lence-causing factors. Canned beans, because they have been cooked at such high temperatures, are the least troublesome, in terms of flatulence, of all beans, except sprouted beans. If you do not want to use canned beans, however, and prefer to cook your own, other ways of reducing their gassiness are to add a couple of pinches of baking soda to the soaking water, or to add ginger, or the Japanese seaweed, kombu.

You can buy digestive enzymes which are specifically designed to help digest beans called alpha-galactosidase, see **Resources**, page 193. You may find it helpful to build up the inclusion of beans in your diet slowly in order to avoid excessive flatulence problems. Start by eating no more than a tablespoon daily and gradually increase the amount to a cup daily. As our digestive tracts respond to the type of meals eaten, you will probably begin to produce the right sort of enzymes over time, as your system has been reminded of the need to do so.

Sprouted beans

By far the best way to neutralise most of the indigestible components is to sprout the legumes before cooking them, this also applies to seeds and grains. All types of beans can be sprouted, as can seeds and grains. By sprouting them you unleash their 'plant-potential' and transform them into vegetables rather than plants-in-waiting. This radically changes their chemistry and increases their nutrient levels. The advantage for anyone with wind problems which are triggered by beans is that they can be transformed in the kitchen into many familiar dishes after they are sprouted. For example, you can make hummus using uncooked sprouted chickpeas, and you can bake bread with sprouted grains. You can also add sprouted beans to soups and stews as you would unsprouted ones. If you are really enthusiastic, you can make delicious biscuits from sprouted grains in special dehydrators, instead of in the oven, which ensures that they retain their full nutritional value. Preparing beans in this way also benefits people who wish to food-combine, as they then become a neutral, non-protein, non-carbohydrate food, see Stop Foods Fighting, page 129.

How to sprout beans

You can sprout any type of dried, whole beans, seeds and grains, although different varieties take differing amounts of time. Mung beans, for instance, only take about three or four days, while chickpeas can take six to seven days. In a clean, wide-necked jar, soak your beans in cooled boiled water, then cover with kitchen paper or muslin secured with an elastic band, and leave in a dark warm place, such as an airing cupboard. Change the water twice a day. Once they begin to sprout, rinse the beans, but return them to the jar damp, not swimming in water. Rinse them twice a day. When the sprouts are long enough, put the jar on a windowsill to catch the sun and enable the sprouted leaves to go slightly green. Your sprouts are ready to eat, and now have more nutrients in them than when you started!

OTHER FOODS THAT PROMOTE GOOD BACTERIA

Cabbage I have already mentioned cabbage in relation to healing the gut wall. It also has the effect of selectively feeding *Lactobacteria*, can suppress the putrefactive bacteria and reduce mucus levels. In order to avoid eating the 450 g a day that is needed to have a marked effect, it is easier to drink 115 ml of cabbage juice twice a day, as described previously. An even more effective way of eating cabbage to promote healthy bowel bacteria is to eat sauerkraut, which is fermented and has already produced lactic acid.

Jerusalem Artichokes These root vegetables are no relation to globe artichokes, but when they are prepared have a similar taste – hence the name. The compound they contain, in large quantities, is called inulin, which is not digested and arrives intact in the bowels to feed colonies of *Lactobacteria* which thrive on it. Just 75–100 g daily can significantly enhance the growth of healthy bacteria. There are two drawbacks to Jerusalem artichokes, however. They also produce large amounts of carbon dioxide which, while it is odourless, can be very uncomfortable for some people. The other drawback is that they can also aggravate candida, if it is present. Theoretically, if you have followed the four-step programme, you will have dealt with any candida at the beginning, but it is something to bear in mind if you are susceptible to the problem.

Onions One large onion eaten daily, cooked or raw, helps to enhance *Lactobacteria* growth. Onions are a beneficial source of many other health producing compounds, including the sulphur amino acids which help to detoxify many compounds.

Yoghurt Live yoghurt is a valuable source of beneficial bacteria and can often be tolerated even by those with a lactose intolerance (though if you do have a lactose intolerance it is best to avoid commercially produced yoghurt). You can add yoghurt to sweet or savoury dishes, or eat it for break-fast or as a snack. If you cook with it, add it to a dish at the last moment to make a creamy sauce. If you add it too early, not only is it likely to curdle, but the heat will destroy the beneficial bacteria.

Now you are home and dry! You have Banished Bloating, and are feeling energetic and healthy. What now? The temptation for some people will be to go back to their old eating patterns. This may not happen overnight, but it is easy, when not following a specific regime, to slide slowly and almost imperceptibly back into familiar habits.

The trick is not to recreate the vicious cycle by again over-doing foods which are likely to induce bloating by damaging the digestive tract wall, or lead to an imbalance in bowel bacteria and an increase in mucus. Generally speaking, this means eating foods to which you are sensitive only on a minimal basis – maybe a couple of times a week. Don't completely deny yourself the pleasure, if this is what it is, just keep these foods for high days and holidays. You should by now have a varied range of substitutes which will, hopefully, have become second nature. You may also find that some of the foods to which you were sensitive have become secondary to any main sensitivities. So, for instance, if previously citrus fruit caused symptoms such as acidity in the stomach or mucus build up in the nasal passages, you may now find that you can happily tolerate orange juice if wheat is kept to a minimum – because the real problem was the wheat, not the orange juice.

The main foods to avoid, which undermine most people with health problems, are refined and sugary foods, excess alcohol (more than one measure a day), gluten grains, dairy products and caffeine containing foods. Keep to a rotation plan for these, while maintaining a high level of fibre, fruit and vegetables in the diet, and you should find that you do not re-establish bloating once it has been banished.

If you do find that you go significantly off the rails, console yourself with the knowledge that it is much easier getting back on track than it is starting from scratch. This is because you will be familiar with what suits you and with food buying and preparation. Sometimes inertia sets in and it seems like an uphill struggle to get going again. The easiest way to deal with this is to focus your mind on a one- or two-week holiday, literal or at home, where you devote time to pampering yourself. During this time you can indulge in a 'cleanse' when you eat and drink in a pure way. Usually at the end of such a period, people find that they remember how great they feel when they follow such a positive eating plan and they find that they do not want to slide back quite so badly into old ways.

A quick checklist of healthy eating options which can help to keep you healthy and bloating-free.

Instead of	Enjoy
Sugar, syrup, honey	Naturally sweet fruits, dried fruits, FOS
White flour, white rice	Brown rice and brown rice flour, buckwheat noodles and flour
Foods to which you are sensitive, such as wheat, dairy, yeast	Refer to the list of alternatives on pages 115, 112 and 136
Salt, highly salted foods	Seaweed flakes, low-salt alternatives, spices, herbs
Saturated and hydrogenated fats	Extra-virgin olive oil, cold pressed flax, sunflower, walnut or sesame oils, nut spreads
Red meat	Fish, organic chicken, game, tofu and other soya products

Instead of	Enjoy
Coffee, strong tea	Dandelion, chicory or other coffee substitutes, herbal or fruit teas
Alcohol	Iced herbal teas, vegetable juices, or alternate each glass of alcohol with a larger glass of water
Colas	Still water mixed with fruit juices

My hope is that you will not feel deprived eating in this way and that you will not feel the need to rebel at the first opportunity. By now your tastes, reactions to foods and attitude to eating will hopefully have been re-educated to appreciate foods which suit your constitution and are health-promoting. Wholefoods, of which there are a huge variety, are far superior in taste terms when compared to pre-packaged foods. Sugary foods really do begin to taste too sweet. The jarring effect of tea or coffee, when avoided for a while, tells its own tale. And the preparation of food really can be enjoyable and not a chore. If you are determined to enjoy the process of understanding your reactions to foods, then you are in the right frame of mind to eat in a way that suits you for the rest of your life.

Part Seven

APPENDICES

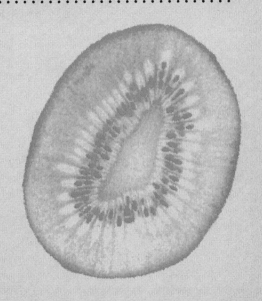

Four-day Planner

You can use this chart when keeping a food diary to work out which foods may be causing problems, or when doing an avoidance and reintroduction test. Feel free to photocopy this page as needed. Record all foods, drinks, times consumed and circumstances (i.e. rushed, relaxed, anxious). You can also use this chart to help plan your meals.

DAY 1	TIME	CIRCUMSTANCES
Breakfast:		
Mid-am:		
Lunch:		
Mid-pm:		
Dinner		
Late snack:		

Any adverse reactions experienced and when:

DAY 2	TIME	CIRCUMSTANCES
Breakfast:		
Mid-am:		
Lunch:		
Mid-pm:		
Dinner		
Late snack:		

Any adverse reactions experienced and when:

DAY 3	TIME	CIRCUMSTANCES
Breakfast:		
Mid-am:		
Lunch:		
Mid-pm:		
Dinner		
Late snack:		

Any adverse reactions experienced and when:

DAY 4	TIME	CIRCUMSTANCES
Breakfast:		
Mid-am:		
Lunch:		
Mid-pm:		
Dinner		
Late snack:		

Any adverse reactions experienced and when:

Suggested Supplement Plan

I have given you many options, throughout the book, of tried and tested solutions to health problems which can lead to bloating. Some readers may feel a little overwhelmed by the sheer volume of different types of supplements, so here is a basic programme which will suit most people and go a long way towards resolving bloating problems. All supplements should be taken daily.

CORE PROGRAMME

1. A good quality multivitamin and multimineral supplement from one of the companies listed in **Resources**, page 193.
2. 2 g vitamin C – preferably with bioflavanoids.

BASIC DIGESTIVE PROGRAMME

3. Digestive enzymes and/or HCl (hydrochloric acid) supplements, if needed (see notes regarding HCl supplements in **Aid Digestion**, page 144).
4. EITHER
   5-10 gms L-glutamine, with vitamin A (7,500 ius in addition to 7,500 ius in the multivitamin) and zinc (10 mg in addition to the 10-15 mg in the multivitamin).
   OR
   Ultraclear Sustain (from Nutri, see **Resources**, page 194)

OR

Enteroguard (from Biocare, see **Resources**, page 193)

FOLLOW-UP PHASE

5. *Acidophilus/Bifidobacteria* supplements
6. FOS (fructo-oligosaccharides) 10 g, and either ground linseeds or psylium husks (see page 169 for details).

The above represents a basic regime. It does not take into account specific problems, such as a candida overgrowth or parasites. It will, however, benefit most people. These supplements should not be taken if you are pregnant, and if you have a medically diagnosed ailment they should not be taken without your doctor's knowledge.

Shopping List

You can use this as a shopping list when becoming familiar with the different products available. It also gives an indication of how many products there are, and just how easy it is to make the transition, say, to a gluten-free diet. A couple of lines have been left at the end of each category for you to add your own products as and when you discover them. Feel free to copy the list as needed.

COW'S MILK ALTERNATIVES

c/l = check label	DAIRY FREE	WHEAT FREE	GLUTEN FREE	NO ADDED SUGARS
Cheese, goat's milk	–	✓	✓	✓
Cheese, sheep's milk	–	✓	✓	✓
Cheese, soya	✓	✓	✓	c/l
Coconut milk	✓	✓	✓	–
Milk, goat's	–	✓	✓	✓
Milk, oat	✓	✓	✓	✓
Milk, rice	✓	✓	✓	✓
Milk, sheep's	–	✓	✓	✓
Milk, soya	✓	✓	✓	c/l
Yoghurt, goat's milk	–	✓	✓	c/l
Yoghurt, sheep's milk	–	✓	✓	c/l
Yoghurt, soya	✓	–	–	c/l

GRAINS AND LEGUMES

c/l = check label	DAIRY FREE	WHEAT FREE	GLUTEN FREE	NO ADDED SUGARS
Beans or lentils canned	✓	✓	✓	c/l
Beans, dried	✓	✓	✓	✓
Bread, sprouted wheat	✓	–	–	–
Bread, pumpernickel	✓	c/l	c/l	–
Bread, 100 per cent rye, raised	✓	✓	–	–
Bread, 100 per cent rye, dark, flat	✓	✓	–	–
Bread 100 per cent rye, sourdough	✓	✓	–	–
Bread, wheat, organic	✓	–	–	–
Bread, wheat, spelt	✓	–	–	–
Cereal, muesli, sugar-free	✓	–	–	✓
Cereal, puffed millet	✓	✓	✓	–
Cereal, puffed quinoa	✓	✓	✓	✓
Cereal, puffed brown rice	✓	✓	✓	c/l
Cereal, puffed wheat, sugar-free	✓	–	–	✓
Cereal, cornflakes, sugar-free	✓	–	–	malted
Crackers, oatcakes	✓	c/l	–	c/l
Crackers, rice cakes	✓	✓	✓	✓
Crackers, rye	✓	c/l	–	✓
Flour, buckwheat	✓	✓	✓	✓
Flour, rice	✓	✓	✓	✓
Flour, rye	✓	✓	–	✓
Flour, spelt	✓	–	–	✓
Flour, gluten-free	✓	✓	✓	✓
Grain, buckwheat	✓	✓	✓	✓
Grain, bulgar wheat (couscous)	✓	–	–	✓

c/l = check label	DAIRY FREE	WHEAT FREE	GLUTEN FREE	NO ADDED SUGARS
Grain, millet	✓	✓	✓	✓
Grain, rice, brown	✓	✓	✓	✓
Oats, flapjacks or biscuits	c/l	✓	–	–
Oats, porridge	✓	✓	–	✓
Pasta, noodles, buckwheat	✓	✓	✓	✓
Pasta, corn	✓	✓	✓	✓
Pasta, rice	✓	✓	✓	✓
Pizza bases, gluten-free	✓	✓	✓	✓
Popadums	✓	c/l	c/l	–
Popcorn, home-made from pack	✓	✓	✓	c/l

SNACKS

c/l = check label	DAIRY FREE	WHEAT FREE	GLUTEN FREE	NO ADDED SUGARS
Fruit, dried, unsulphured	✓	✓	✓	✓
Fruit, bars	c/l	c/l	c/l	c/l
Muesli, bars	c/l	c/l	c/l	c/l
Nuts, raw, unsalted	✓	✓	✓	✓
Olives	✓	✓	✓	✓
Rice, Chinese snacks	✓	✓	✓	c/l
Seeds, raw, unsalted	✓	✓	✓	✓
Sesame snaps	✓	✓	✓	–
Sesame sticks	✓	✓	✓	✓

FATS, OILS, SPREADS

c/l = check label	DAIRY FREE	WHEAT FREE	GLUTEN FREE	NO ADDED SUGARS
Emulsified margarines (Vitaquel/Granose)	✓	✓	✓	✓
Soya margarine	✓	✓	✓	✓
Extra virgin olive oil	✓	✓	✓	✓
Essential balance oil	✓	✓	✓	✓
Flax seed oil	✓	✓	✓	✓
Sunflower seed butter	✓	✓	✓	✓
Cashew nut butter	✓	✓	✓	✓
Almond nut butter	✓	✓	✓	✓

DRINKS

c/l = check label	DAIRY FREE	WHEAT FREE	GLUTEN FREE	NO ADDED SUGARS
Caro	✓	✓	–	✓
Barleycup	✓	✓	–	✓
Dandelion coffee	–	✓	✓	–
Herb and fruit teas	✓	✓	✓	✓
Aqualibra	✓	✓	✓	✓
Amé	✓	✓	✓	✓

MISCELLANEOUS

c/l = check label	DAIRY FREE	WHEAT FREE	GLUTEN FREE	NO ADDED SUGARS
Seaweeds, condiments	✓	✓	✓	✓
Seeds, linseeds	✓	✓	✓	✓
Sweetener, fructose	✓	✓	✓	fructose
Sweetener, honey	✓	✓	✓	fructose/ glucose
Tamari, wheat-free soya sauce	✓	✓	✓	✓
Tofu, soya	✓	✓	✓	✓

Resources

If you wish to be kept informed of Suzannah Olivier's books, workshops and other activities visit her website: www.healthandnutrition.co.uk or E-mail: eattobefit@aol.com

SUPPLEMENT COMPANIES

BIOCARE Birmingham, Tel: 0121 433 3727
- Stocked by good independent health food shops. Direct mail ordering service available.
- Nutrients: large range of vitamins, minerals and essential fats. Mixed Ascorbates is a good powdered buffered vitamin C with flavanoids.
- Fibre: Colon Care.
- Liver support: HEP 194.
- Oedema: celery seed extract.
- Digestive enzymes: range of digestive enzymes. An excellent general one is Polyzyme Forte, others are specific to people who have problems with digesting specific food groups, i.e. carbohydrates, gluten, milk, lactose, fats.
- Anti-microbial/anti-parasitic: Garlic Plus, Biocidin (grapefruit seed), Artemisia complex, Oregano Complex (micellised plant oils) and other of formula preparations such as Eradacidin Forte (grapefruit seed extract, Artemisia and berberis), Candistatin (contains Pau d'Arco).
- Pre/pro-biotics: FOS, Fructo-lite (liquid FOS), a range of acidophilus products, including Replete which is an intensive, seven-day, intestinal recolonisation programme, particularly useful after antibiotic use.
- Intestinal conditioners: Butyric Acid complex, NAG, Enteroguard (for leaky gut), Gastroplex (gamma oryzanol, slippery elm and marshmallow), Muccolyte.

HIGHER NATURE East Sussex, Tel: 01435 882880
- Direct mail ordering service available.
- Nutrients: range of vitamins, minerals and essential fats. They also supply flax seed oil and essential balance oil which are excellent alternatives to other salad oils.
- Fibre: Colofibre*, Hi-lignan (flax seed powder).

- Liver support: Liverite (animal based).
- Digestive enzymes: Easigest, Betaine HCl.
- Pre/pro-biotics: FOS, Lactogest, Acidobifidus, Probiogest.
- Anti-microbials/anti-parasitic: colloidal silver, Citricidal (liquid or tablet form of grapefruit seed extract), Herbal Clear, Paracleans.
- Intestinal conditioner: L-glutamine, aloe vera, Coloclear*, Cat's Claw Tea.

  * Colofibre, Coloclear plus Herbal Clear make an excellent colon cleansing programme.

LAMBERTS Kent, Tel: 01892 552120

- Available from health clinics and pharmacies.
- Nutrients: large range of vitamins, minerals and essential fats.
- Fibre: Colon-cleanse (contains apple fibre and a selection of herbs such as fennel, black walnut, milk thistle, dandelion root, red clover).
- Liver support: milk thistle.
- Digestive enzymes: Digestizyme®, Betaine HCl with Pepsin.
- Anti-microbial/anti-parasitic: garlic/Pure-Gar®.
- Pre/pro-biotics: Acidophilus Extra, Eliminex® (FOS).
- Intestinal conditioner: aloe vera capsules, L-glutamine.

NUTRI High Peak, Tel: 0800 212742

- Nutrients: large range of vitamins, minerals and essential fats.
- Fibre: fibre formula, GastroCleanse (ophilus).
- Liver support: Detoxification Factors multivitamin and mineral, Ultra Clear, Ultra Clear Plus.
- Digestive enzymes: Similase and Hypo-D.
- Anti-microbial/anti-parasitic: they have an excellent herbal formula called ParaGuard. Exspore (an anti-candida formula which includes grapefruit seed extract, Pau d'arco, cloves, golden seal and caprylic acid).
- Pre/pro-biotics: Enterogenic Concentrate.
- Intestinal conditioner: Gastric complex (contains gamma oryzanol, mashmallow and slippery elm), Gut Permeability Factors and Ultra Clear Sustain. Ultra Clear Sustain is a meal replacement powder, which is consumed as a drink. It contains vitamins, minerals and amino acids that support the liver, help heal the digestive tract and support the growth of friendly bacteria.

THE NUTRI CENTRE London W1, Tel: 020 7436 5122

- Stock a wide range of nutrition products, health foods and books from various suppliers and manufacturers. They also supply the NutriWest range. You can either visit the shop or obtain their products by mail order.

SOLGAR Herts, Tel: 01442 890355
- Stocked by good independent health food shops.
- Nutrients: large range of low to high dose vitamins, minerals and essential fats.
- Fibre: Psyllium, apple pectin, multi-fibre formula.
- Liver support: milk thistle and dandelion herbal complex and milk thistle.
- Digestive enzymes: digestive enzymes (general formula), Vegan Formula Digestive Aid, Betaine HCl, Lactase.
- Anti-microbial/anti-parasitic: Golden Seal, garlic, Pau d'Arco.
- Pre/pro-biotics: range of acidophilus supplements.
- Intestinal conditioners: L-glutamine, alfalfa, aloe vera, cayenne (mild stimulant).

BEST CARE PRODUCTS East Sussex, Tel: 01342 410303
www.bestcare-uk.com
- Supply herbal supplement programmes for detoxification and digestive health.

BIONAL UK LTD London SW8, Tel: 0800 328 4244
- Cream and supplements for puffy legs. Stocked in health food shops.

XYNERGY Tel: 01730 813642
- Lifestream Biogenic Aloe Vera, as well as an excellent range of 'green' foods (algae, spirulina, etc). Direct mail ordering service available.

ENZYME PROCESS Tel: 01775 761927
- For a superb range of enzymes.

BLACKMORES
- In good quality health food shops. A full range of good quality herbs for every need.

SIMMONDS HERBAL SUPPLIES East Sussex, Tel: 0800 542 5212
www.herbalsupplies.com
- An superb range of herbal products available by mail order.

HOW TO FIND A NUTRITIONAL THERAPIST OR DOCTOR

BRITISH ASSOCIATION OF NUTRITIONAL THERAPISTS (BANT) London SE13, Tel: 0181 692 1398
INSTITUTE FOR OPTIMUM NUTRITION (ION) London SW5, Tel: 0181 877 9993
List of qualified nutritionists (small cost) and training courses.
BRITISH SOCIETY FOR ALLERGY AND ENVIRONMENTAL MEDICINE (BAESNM) Southampton, Tel: 01703 812 124
For a list of medical doctors who have a particular interest in nutritional medicine.

BIOCHEMICAL TESTING

Most of these tests are available only through practitioners. If you do obtain one direct you are strongly advised to get it interpreted by a nutritionist or other qualified health professional so that the results of the test can be acted on appropriately. While these tests can be of use (particularly the gut permeability and CDSA tests) please see the relevant sections of the book for their limitations.

BRAMPTOM SCIENTIFIC SERVICES FOOD ALLERGY/INTOLERANCE TESTING Tel: 01582 883014
Postal tests available.

DIAGNOSTECH LTD Swansea, Tel: 0800 731 5655
Tests include: Candiscan, their test for candida albicans, female hormone profile and adrenal stress.

DIAGNOSTIC SERVICES LTD Liverpool, Tel: 0151 922 6200
Part of the Nutri group, High Peak. Blood screening tests include: thyroid profile, liver profile and renal (kidney) profile.

GREAT SMOKIES DIAGNOSTIC LABORATORY
The services of this laboratory can be organised through their UK agents, Diagnostic Services Ltd, Tel: 0151 922 6200.
Their non-invasive tests include: comprehensive digestive stool analysis, detoxification profile, parasitology, candida, *Helicobacter pylori*, intestinal permeability, lactose intolerance breath test. Postal service.

INDIVIDUAL WELLBEING DIAGNOSTIC LABORATORY
London SW3, Tel: 0171 730 7010
Tests include: allergy and food additive intolerance (FACT), *Helicobacter pylori*, adrenal stress index, gluten and candida. Has a clinic as well as a postal service. All tests are supported by a nutritional consultation.

UNI-KEY HEALTH SYSTEMS Bozeman, Montana, USA, Tel: 001 406 587 6701
Mail order parasite test kit.

YORK NUTRITIONAL LABORATORY York, Tel: 0800 074 6185
Food intolerance and allergy testing. Postal service.

ORGANIC FOOD SOURCES

THE SOIL ASSOCIATION Bristol House, 40-56 Victoria Street, Bristol BS1 6BY Tel: 0117 929 0661
The Soil Association can provide a list of organic suppliers in the UK, as well as publications on organic issues. Telephone to check the price of the catalogue.

GLUTEN FREE FOODS

INTERNET MAIL ORDER
www.glutenfree-foods.co.uk
www.realhealth.co.uk

TERRANCE STAMP FOODS
All-purpose flour, vegetable crisps, wheat free pasta, etc.
Manufactured by Buxton Foods. Available from some selected super-
markets (Waitrose, Sainsburys, Safeways) and health food stores.

KJAERS FOOD FOR LIFE The Village Bakery Melmesbury Ltd, Penrith,
Cumbria, CA10 1HE
Gluten free bread, cakes and biscuits. Write to them for a list of
stockists.

WHOLISTIC RESEARCH CO LTD Tel: 01707 262 686
www.wholisticresearch.com The Old Forge, Mill Green, Hatfield, Herts,
AL9 5NZ
Grain sprouters, dehydrators, water distillers, juicers.

ASSOCIATIONS

BRITISH DIGESTIVE FOUNDATION
Free information leaflets. Send an SAE to PO Box 251, Edgware,
Middlesex, HA8 6HG

IBS NETWORK Tel: 0114 261 1531
It costs £15 to join the IBS network, which includes a quarterly journal
Gut Reaction, access to 'befrienders', a telephone hotline, self-help
groups and therapeutic courses.

COELIACS SOCIETY P.O. Box 220, High Wycombe, Bucks, HP11 2HY
To request information about Coeliacs disease send an SAE.

Other Associations

COLONICS INTERNATIONAL ASSOCIATION (CIA) Tel: 01442
827687 16 Drumond Ride, Tring, Herts, HP23 5DE
For a list of registered therapists who practise colonic irrigation send
an SAE.

ASSOCIATION OF SYSTEMATIC KINESIOLOGY Surbiton, Tel:
0181 399 3215
To find a qualified therapist in kinesiology.

KINESIOLOGY FEDERATION Knebworth, Tel: 01438 817998
email: kinesiology@btinternet.net

BOOKS

Gluten Free, Dairy Free and Allergy Management Cook Books

Allergy Free Eating Michelle Berridale-Johnson, Thorsons, 1999
Allergy Free Eating Liz Reno and Joanna Derais, Celestial Arts, USA, 1992, reprinted 1995
Cooking Without Barbara Cousins, Thorsons, 1997
The Stamp Collection Terrence Stamp, Ebury, 1998

Stress Management Books

Emotional Cleaning John Ruskan, Rider, 1998
Feel the Fear and Do It Anyway Susan Jeffers, Arrow, 1996
Out of Pain into Power Bill Longridge, Rider, 1999
The Stress Protection Plan Suzannah Olivier, Collins & Brown, 2000

Specific Diet Books

Breaking the Vicious Cycle Elaine Gottschall, Kirkton Press, Canada, 1994, reprinted 1996
Digestive Wellness Elizabeth Lipski, Keats, USA, 1996
Eat Right 4 Your Type Peter d'Adamo, Random House, 1998
Erica White's Beat Candida Cookbook Erica White, Thorsons, 1999
Food Combining for Health Doris Grant and Jean Joyce, Thorsons, 1991
Food Combining for Vegetarians Jackie Le Tissier, Thorsons, 1992

Other Books of Interest

Digestive Enzymes Jeffrey Bland, Keats Publishing, USA, 1986
Genetic Nutritionering Jeffrey Bland, Keats Incorp, USA, 1999